OF CANCER AND MARATHONS

OF CANCER AND MARATHONS

THE RUN OF A LIFETIME

SHIRAZ SIDDIQUI

AMARYLLIS

AMARYLLIS
An imprint of Manjul Publishing House Pvt. Ltd.
• C-16, Sector 3, Noida, Uttar Pradesh 201301, India
Website: www.manjulindia.com
Registered Office:
• 2nd Floor, Usha Preet Complex, 42 Malviya Nagar, Bhopal 462 003 – India
Distribution Centres
Ahmedabad, Bengaluru, Bhopal, Chennai, Hyderabad,
Kolkata, Mumbai, Noida, Pune

Of Cancer and Marathons: The Run of a Lifetime by Shiraz Siddiqui

This paperback edition first published in India in 2024

ISBN 978-93-5543-336-7

Printed and bound in India by Parksons Graphics Pvt. Ltd.

The content of this book is the sole expression and opinion of its author and not that of the publisher. The medical diagnosis and line of treatment are specific to the author's ailment as were offered by medical experts. These are not intended for use, in any manner, by the general public. The author or the publisher will not be liable, monetarily or otherwise, for any unauthorized usage of any of the contents of this book.

Contents

FOREWORD I

I LIKED HIS SIMPLE, SCIENTIFIC APPROACH

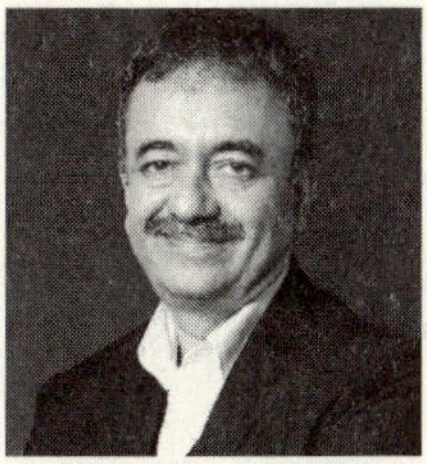

Rajkumar Hirani
Filmmaker, Director, Producer

In our growing-up years, I remember never giving importance to any kind of physical exercise. As you grow older, you feel the body needs more attention. Way back in 2014, I reached out to a friend who I thought took good care of his body and was aware of fitness theories. He made me meet Shiraz.

During our first meeting, I realised that Shiraz was not only a professional nutritionist and a wellness coach but also a cancer survivor who bravely fought two relapses and a bone marrow transplant and was aiming to complete the 90-kilometre Comrades race. Looking at him I could not make out that he had been through chemotherapy and fought the cancer battle twice. He looked so fit.

Apart from an exclusive style of training, I was impressed with the vast knowledge and well-defined scientific approach to health and wellness that he had to offer, from advising me to do a series of pathological tests to doing a genetic analysis. Our journey started with understanding my physical strength, weaknesses and imbalances in my body.

Shiraz's approach was very simple—he not only believed in clean eating but also wanted his clients to understand every aspect of nutrition. This approach to fitness and nutrition not only helped me but also my family in achieving good health with a simple philosophy that whatever you start with, you should continue it for life and make it your lifestyle so that you enjoy doing it.

I'm happy that he has written a book and shared his life knowledge with all. I wish him the best… Always.

FOREWORD II

INSPIRING OUR SON FROM PASSION TO PODIUM

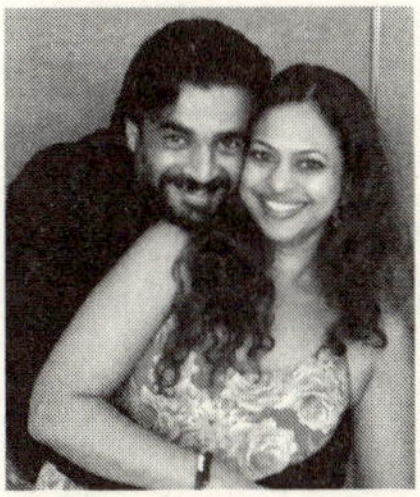

Sarita & R Madhavan
R Madhavan's wife | Film Actor, Writer, Filmmaker, Producer

In 2018, when our son Vedaant won his first international medal in swimming—a bronze in the 1500m freestyle—at the Thailand Age Group Swimming Championship, we were filled with an overwhelming sense of pride as parents. It was a moment of pure joy, knowing that we had supported our son in pursuing his passion. Little did we know that this was just the beginning of an incredible journey that would shape Vedaant's future.

With each subsequent competition, Vedaant's collection of medals grew, cementing his position as a rising star in the world of swimming. Today, he stands before us as a beacon of hope, a promising contender for an Olympic medal, proudly representing India.

Throughout this remarkable journey, there was one individual who played an instrumental role in Vedaant's success—Shiraz.

Shiraz possessed an exceptional talent for crafting personalised diet plans that perfectly complement Vedaant's unique lifestyle. As Vedaant's parents, our primary concern is not only our child's success but also his overall well-being, and for this, we are immensely grateful to Shiraz.

Shiraz also had a profound understanding of Vedaant's specific dietary requirements, a quality that distinguished him from others as an inspiring figure. He empowered others to maintain focus and prioritise their health without resorting to potentially harmful supplements. Under Shiraz's expert guidance, Vedaant made extraordinary progress in an astonishingly short period, blossoming into a swimming champion, and garnering numerous accolades along the way.

However, what set Shiraz apart from others was not just his exceptional skill in nutrition, but also his unwavering spirit and determination in the face of adversity. Despite battling cancer, Shiraz displayed incredible resilience and became a true fighter. His unwavering commitment to his health and well-being serves as a remarkable inspiration to us all.

It is awe-inspiring to witness how, despite his ailment, Shiraz managed to establish a fitness company of such high repute. His ability to overcome personal challenges and channelise his energy into helping others achieve their fitness goals was truly commendable. Shiraz's story serves as a testament to the power of determination and the triumph of the human spirit.

We have had the privilege of working with Shiraz, who not only excelled in his field but also served as a living embodiment of strength and resilience. His knowledge, dedication and steady determination were qualities that made him an exceptional role model.

Shiraz's resolute commitment to his craft and his inspiring fight against cancer are deserving of immense praise and recognition. Shiraz's story reminds us that no matter the obstacles we face, with determination and perseverance, we can achieve greatness.

INTRODUCTION

It was the year 2003, and I was just twenty-seven years old, brimming with vitality and strength. As a dedicated fitness instructor at JW Marriott in Mumbai, I had the privilege of imparting my knowledge to high-net-worth individuals (HNIs), guiding them towards a healthy lifestyle. With five years of experience in the fitness industry, I garnered immense respect and became a much-sought-after professional due to my qualifications as a nutritionist, martial arts practitioner and accomplished marathon runner. It fills my heart with pride to say that my robust health was so unwavering that I had never required a single paracetamol tablet in my entire life!

Growing up in the challenging environment of Saki Naka, Mumbai, was no easy feat, but my profession alleviated my family's financial struggles. The prospect of a bright future awaited me, alongside my loving Ammi (mother), Abbu (father) and brother Firoz. I yearned for greater achievements, financial prosperity, a joyous marriage and a life of comfort.

However, fate had other plans in store for me—plans I was wholly unaware of at the time. In 2004, I was unexpectedly confronted with a devastating diagnosis: Acute Lymphoblastic Leukaemia (A.L.L.), a form of blood cancer notorious for granting its victims a mere five years of survival, if lucky enough to experience remission at all. Yet, my journey was far from the ordinary. I defied the stringent confines of the five-year deadline imposed by this merciless disease.

Armed with unwavering determination and drawing strength from my martial arts and fitness training, I fearlessly battled the cancer with all my might. Astonishingly, my resilience yielded miraculous results—I not only achieved one but two successful remissions! Additionally, I underwent a bone marrow transplant, an arduous procedure that caused my blood's RH factor to alter thrice, resulting in my living with three distinct blood groups!

Nevertheless, cancer was not yet finished with its relentless assault on my body. I encountered two subsequent relapses, each introducing different forms of cancer. There were moments when excruciating pain rendered me unable to walk or eat, driving me to scream in sheer frustration. The disease depleted my hard-earned savings, drained my energy and mercilessly ravaged my once-vibrant physique.

Yet, in the depths of my struggle, gratitude enveloped my spirit. I am eternally grateful to the human beings who came to me as angels during my darkest hours, offering invaluable financial assistance, sacrificing their precious time, and providing solace and unyielding support. They became the pillars that held me when I reached the nadir of my existence, propelling me forward on my path to recovery.

Their unwavering dedication enabled me to rise from the ashes and establish my own fitness company, which swiftly became a go-to training centre for HNIs, employing over thirty passionate individuals.

Furthermore, it allowed me to reignite my passion for running marathons, initially participating in half marathons and ultimately achieving an awe-inspiring record in a full one. I even had the privilege of competing on national and international stages, while my company inspired countless individuals to embrace a fitness-driven lifestyle and participate in marathons themselves.

I consider myself extraordinarily blessed to possess the training and indomitable willpower necessary to safeguard myself from the clutches of cancer. Moreover, I cherish the profound lessons this relentless battle has bestowed upon me. My story has confounded medical professionals and defied the boundaries of conventional medical records, and my ability to bounce back each time has filled me with immense pride and a profound sense of accomplishment.

Furthermore, my life is graced by the presence of an incredible woman, my beloved wife, Nida. She has remained steadfast by my side through thick and thin, offering unwavering support during the most challenging periods of my treatments and even running marathons alongside me, a living testament to her unmatched devotion.

My ultimate dream remains unchanged—to participate in the prestigious Comrades Marathon, The Ultimate Human Race, a gruelling ultramarathon held annually in South Africa. For years, I meticulously planned and prepared for this monumental event, hoping to participate during a brief period of respite from cancer. However, as fate would have it, my aspirations were cruelly shattered by the unforeseen arrival of the COVID-19 pandemic. Last year seemed to present a glimmer of hope, but alas, the Big C dealt another painful blow, and I experienced a heart-wrenching relapse.

Nevertheless, I adamantly refuse to surrender. I am steadily recovering, rising once again, and mustering the courage to fight back, confident that I will soon conquer the Comrades, fulfilling the promise I made to myself.

As the legendary boxer Muhammad Ali so eloquently stated, 'Only a man who knows what it is like to be defeated can reach down to the bottom of his soul and come up with the extra ounce of power it takes to win when the match is even.' Today, as I pen these words, my battle with cancer nears the remarkable milestone of nineteen years. It has been an arduous and profoundly transformative journey, teaching me invaluable lessons along the way.

My utmost desire is for my tale to inspire anyone grappling with health challenges. Whether battling cancer or any other ailment, it is essential to recognise that our mental fortitude plays an unparalleled role in our overall well-being. The physical battle is inevitably intertwined with our mental state; when we lose the battle in our minds, victory in the physical realm becomes increasingly elusive.

The human mind possesses unparalleled power—it has the potential to either heal us or destroy us. It all depends on how we train and harness its capabilities. No matter what the ailment is, we must assume control and refuse to allow it to dominate our lives.

Through meticulous research, conversations with medical professionals and self-understanding, I endeavoured to comprehend the intricacies of my ailment. I delved into medical research, evaluating the effects they had on my body, and conscientiously curated a diet that countered the accompanying side effects. Vigilantly monitoring my body's responses to various stimuli became an integral part of my healing journey, and my background as a nutritionist played a pivotal role in this process.

Ultimately, the closer we come to understanding our bodies, the more equipped we become to confront the challenges that life throws our way. Yes, there were countless moments when I felt utterly defeated, crying out to God with a resounding 'Why me?', a seething rage bubbling within, a palpable sense of helplessness. At times, I contemplated surrender, questioning if this marked the culmination of my existence.

Yet, in those dire moments, my disciplined mind emerged as a guiding light. It propelled me forward, nurturing the resilience necessary to triumph and embrace a new day. Today, I earnestly hope that my journey will ignite a spark of inspiration within you, empowering you to surmount your obstacles. I have also extensively elaborated on how I prepared for my marathons, and I hope it makes you want to run too!

Thank you for taking out time to listen to my story, and I fervently wish you strength and triumph on your unique path of resilience.

PART I

You don't know what life has in store for you, but it prepares you in its unique way

1

LIFE WAS TOUGH, BUT IT WAS GOOD

The Lilavati Hospital and Medical Centre, a luxurious five-star medical facility nestled in the peaceful neighbourhood of Bandra, is a popular choice for Mumbai's elite. With an outstanding team of doctors, efficient medical services, and a serene atmosphere, it's easy to see why. The rooms provide a breathtaking view of the Arabian Sea and the charming Bandra bungalows, offering a temporary escape from life's worries. However, my experience was far from enjoyable.

I was confined to my eighth-floor isolation 'box', undergoing chemotherapy, feeling isolated both physically and spiritually. I wondered when I would be free from this imprisonment. It was November 2004, and I reflected on the unexpected turn my life had taken. I had always been a happy-go-lucky guy, in love with jogging. The rhythm of my feet hitting the ground gave me a sense of peace, and I never needed anyone. But this was different.

Lilavati Hospital's treatment protocol required isolation to protect my fragile body from infection. What frightened me was not knowing when or if I would ever be able to leave.

Would I ever run again? I was Shiraz Siddiqui, the certified nutritionist and fitness trainer who helped others get in shape. I had never smoked or consumed alcohol my whole life. I always ate healthy and exercised more than necessary. My body was my temple, and I inspired others to follow my example. Despite all this, I had been diagnosed with acute lymphoblastic leukaemia (A.L.L.). How could this happen to me?

'Blood cancer is treatable,' my physicians assured me. 'You need to make lifestyle changes.' However, none of them knew anyone who had survived for more than five years after being diagnosed. I was not ready to give up on life. I was prepared to hold it together with paper clips. During such times, your spirit becomes your sole companion. Conversations with my spirit kept me going.

'Do you still believe in life after all that you've been through?' it asked.

'Of course, I do,' I replied with a stoic smile.

And my spirit smiled back.

Tough, but Enjoyable Childhood

Cancer was just one of many obstacles in my life's journey. Before my diagnosis, I had grown up in a humble abode known as a *chawl*—a linear structure with a shared corridor, a community toilet, a washing area, and a balcony—nestled in the bustling Saki Naka neighbourhood of Mumbai.

Inside our 200-square-foot room lived a family of six: Ammi (my serene warrior mother), Abbu (my ever-busy father), my brother Firoz, two uncles, and me. But despite the tight quarters, our home never felt cramped. My mother's housekeeping skills were second to none, and her pride and joy was the leg-operated Usha sewing machine that sat in the corner. The machine not only provided her with a creative outlet, but the box in which it came doubled up as our dining table when she folded the machine away in it.

The centrepiece of the room was the gleaming two-door Godrej cupboard, which also had a mirror on one side. My mother would often dress up in front of the mirror, mimicking the Bollywood heroines of her youth. She would perfect her most frightening facial expressions, which would come in handy on those nights when the power went out, and the lanterns/candles were lit, and we were left to our imaginations.

The common toilet was my worst nightmare. A friend had warned me of ghosts lurking inside during the night, leaving me so petrified that I often held it in until the morning. Even then, the ordeal of staying up at night was far from over. If not using the bathroom, a chore that needed to be done in the middle of the night was filling up water. Every day, at 3.30 a.m., we would attach a big rubber pipe to the common tap, securing it with a white rope to keep it in place. If the rope came loose, we would have to sprint to the end of the row of houses to fix it again. It was a chaotic affair, with everyone scrambling to fill their containers before water supply was cut off at 5 a.m.

On monsoon days, the house would flood, and water would seep through the walls, making its way into our home. The small bookshelf that held our schoolbooks and prized black-and-white Dyanora TV would need to be propped up on bricks to avoid water damage.

But despite these challenges, we always managed to make ends meet. My parents worked tirelessly to pay for our school fees, books and other necessities, while my brother and I pitched in wherever we could. I longed to be financially independent, but looking back, I am grateful for the lessons in resilience and resourcefulness that I learned from my upbringing.

In 1994, my older brother Firoz bagged a job at Mafatlal. So we left our chawl and moved to a modest pad in far-flung Kalyan. It was time for me to contribute. I took up a trainer's role at a tiny gym in Mulund, but it was a hard gig money-wise. I was looking for another job, but was unable to get anything that had decent pay. My fitness career hit a wall, and I was fretting.

I sent an application to a branch of Talwalkar's Gym in a well-known locality, but they gave me the boot, citing my long commute from Kalyan to Mumbai as a problem. I swore I'd manage it, but they didn't seem convinced. I also tried the gym at the Ramada Palm Grove Hotel, but something about it put me off.

I pinned my hopes on JW Marriott, India's numero uno hotel chain, despite it being in the posh Juhu locality, another Mumbai suburb far from Kalyan. Marriott had advertised in the papers for a fitness coach as they were in the pre-opening phase. I cleared their interview rounds with ease, waiting for the final one when the general manager himself sauntered in and led me to his desk. His courteous behaviour bowled me over. This is the boss I want to work with, I thought to myself.

'How will you make it to Juhu every day from Kalyan?' he asked.

'No sweat, sir,' I said. 'I'll figure something out. If needed, I'll rent a place nearby.'

The offer letter soon arrived, and I became a nutrition and fitness consultant, starting at Rs 5,000 (about $60). It was a dream job, and my heart leapt with joy knowing my family's financial struggles would ease up a bit. Finally, I was self-sufficient, and my mind found peace. This was in 2001.

The next two years were a whirlwind of preparation. Only thirteen of us had the colossal task of prepping up a million square feet of leisure space. We worked tirelessly, putting in double and triple shifts, but each day brought a sense of accomplishment.

Finally, on 31 December 2001, we completed our pre-opening training, and the palatial JW Marriott was set to open its doors in the new year. Standing on the pool deck, with the Arabian Sea roaring behind us, I told my colleagues that this was where we would become the best in our profession. I could feel the salty sea air filling my lungs with joy. 'Here, we will make history,' I said, taking a deep breath.

The first two years at Marriott Juhu flew by. My team and I worked hard to persuade the management of the need to have personalised training packages. Marriott was the first five-star hotel to sell local gym memberships, and it was a massive success. My career also soared, and the few thousand on my pay cheque multiplied by at least ten times to a lakh ($1200) and beyond. Though some of the colleagues who had started off with me had dropped out, those that remained were on a high. Their hard work and determination had paid off.

My life began to settle down. My family moved away from Kalyan, and Ammi and I rented an apartment in Andheri, closer to the Marriott. Firoz began working in Saudi Arabia, and along with his wife, Meher, he purchased a small flat in Thane.

I was at the top of my game, free from struggles and dependence. Finally, Ammi's 'sheru' and Abba's 'sher' could roar. I smiled triumphantly, relishing my newfound freedom. My life and dreams were becoming a reality, or at least that's what it felt like at the time.

2

THE EARLY SYMPTOMS

1 August 2004: My health was deteriorating at this time. I began to feel tired. 'Are the severe cramps in my calves causing me to feel low?' I thought. I resolved to solve the problem. I went in for a CBC (complete blood count) test in the first week of August.

'It's just a drop in haemoglobin. It has decreased from 14.5 to 11.8. Nothing major,' Dr Kalpana Rao, Marriott's in-house doctor, said. 'Anaemia is a simple iron deficiency. Take some shots and load up on iron-rich foods.'

I was feeling better a month later. But something was bothering me. The long hours were getting to me. As a team leader and executive, I'd be in and out of meetings, leading training sessions for the gym and pool teams, and overseeing a team of thirty employees. I was also overbooked as the best trainer on the floor. Personal training was not permitted during shifts, so I would stay afterwards for training and dietary consultations. My stress levels would undoubtedly be high, I reasoned to myself.

My body was screaming for attention. The normally healthy boy was invariably sick with a cold, was frequently feverish and weary. I persuaded myself to repeat the CBC test. This time, the haemoglobin level had plummeted even lower to 10. The white cell count was 3,200, which was a little lower than the normal level of 4,000. Even the platelets were borderline normal.

This time, Dr Kalpana directed me to meet with a Doctor of Medicine (MD). 'It's a typical case of megaloblastic anaemia, folic acid and B12 deficiency,' the doctor explained.

'However, I am a non-vegetarian. I frequently consume eggs, chicken and fish. There is an abundance of B12 in my diet. It's not possible,' I said, the fitness and nutritionist in me not ready to accept the doctor's diagnosis.

But I did as he instructed and took the B12 shots. But they did not help much.

My health deteriorated progressively over the next few months. Based on my appearance and fitness levels, two more doctors dismissed me by saying it was fatigue. But my body was telling me otherwise. I used to be too unwell to go to work on some days. On other days, I couldn't concentrate, needed to sleep frequently, and was dependent on paracetamol for my low-grade temperature.

'At twenty-eight, this is the first time I'm taking medication regularly,' I reflected. I decided to go for another CBC test.

The reports this time were troubling. The haemoglobin level had dropped to nine. The platelets were down to 84,000, compared to the usual 1,50,000.

I was fighting for air as I climbed the one floor to the office. 'And I am the fitness guy,' I grumbled. A part of me was telling me to slow down. However, I pushed that notion aside and resolved to address this health issue. Fast.

I contacted Lilavati Hospital in Mumbai to get an appointment with a haematologist. 'Dr Abhay Bhave is available for consultation. But all his appointments for the day are booked.'

I was on a get-well-soon mission. I went straight to the Lilavati Outpatient Department (OPD) and waited till Dr Bhave's last appointment was attended. When he was set to leave, I requested him to see me as my case was urgent. The courteous man sat and waited, checking my reports, and performing a medical check-up.

'I need you to run a battery of tests to rule out HIV, hepatitis, and any other serious anaemia and blood-related diseases,' the good doctor stated. I submitted my blood samples the same night.

The results of the testing were clear.

'A bone marrow biopsy is required. Bring a guardian with you, and we'll do the rest,' Dr Bhave said.

'I only have an elderly mother. My brother works overseas. I'll have to come alone,' I stated emphatically.

'Will you be okay if we do the biopsy procedure under local anaesthesia?' Dr Bhave inquired.

'That's alright if I can return home the same day, as it's only me and my mother at home,' I informed him. I went home and didn't share anything with Ammi. I felt like a ten-year-old again, who was scared to inform his mother that he had a school test the next day.

The following day I went back to becoming a baby again. I lay down on one side and curled my legs to my chest in a foetal position as instructed. My hip bone was precisely located by the doctor's fingers. I felt the stinging agony of the anaesthetic needle entering the bone. Then everything went numb. Despite the large number of people there, the room with its yellow lighting was quiet. I didn't realise it at the time, but Dr Bhave couldn't aspirate or remove much of my bone marrow. He was now penetrating the bone to obtain a small sample for the histopathologist's biopsy. I could feel the severe pain in the bone even while under local anaesthesia.

Two days later, Dr Bhave called to schedule another bone marrow biopsy.

This time, I was certain I was in big trouble.

The Shocker

Firoz had flown in from Saudi Arabia for a short vacation. 'Go slow, Abrar,' Ammi instructed her five-year-old grandson, while adoringly rocking baby Ayesha. Senior Siddiqui's house was buzzing with the excitement of the family reuniting after a long separation. We brothers decided to go for a walk in the cool evening air.

Dr Bhave's office called. It had been about a fortnight since all the testing had been completed, and the doctor had finally received all his reports. 'It's leukaemia,' Dr Bhave said. 'We need you to come in for an advanced test to determine the stage and type.' I was shell-shocked!

I told Firoz about my entire journey and we immediately went to an internet cafe to do some preliminary research.

My bones have all dried up, I thought, as I prepared to go to the doctor the next day.

The next round of reports arrived. 'It is unequivocally a case of acute lymphoblastic leukaemia (A.L.L.). The blast cells, the cancerous cells, have exceeded 70 per cent,' said Dr Bhave, adding, 'but it is treatable.'

'There is some good news, too,' Dr Bhave added. 'You don't have the Philadelphia strain.'

A strain named after a city in the United States?

'That one is fatal,' Dr Bhave said emphatically.

He spoke like my instructors at Saki Naka's St. Anthony's High School. 'His report card is quite poor. But there is some good news. He's at least talented in sports.'

My mother had not been overjoyed with the news. To her, my treasure trove of a dozen certificates from each Annual Sports Day was just paper. 'Stop collecting *raddi*,' Ammi said. 'You should sell it. It will generate some revenue.' However, my investment in raddi had paid off.

As the first person in my school to learn table tennis, I was invited to a summer camp during my seventh-grade vacations. I'd be the table tennis instructor. It was an incredible honour. I was relieved that Ammi would finally hear some good news. And she did, because my first official job paid me Rs 250 ($3).

I felt like one of those rag-pickers whose life I used to ponder during my early runs before school. Those elderly ladies in paper-thin saris and guys in nothing more than a lungi or a dhoti would be too busy separating plastic, metal, and paper barefoot. Why were these poor people checking out this filth as if they were searching for gold? What if they became sick? I knew nothing about waste management or recycling, but I felt sympathy for them.

Now that I didn't have this Philadelphia strain in my leukaemia, it felt like I'd found the gold in the raddi.

* * *

The ever-practical fitness trainer in me refused to be shaken by the news that I had cancer. It's a major shock, like what I experienced when I failed four of my preliminary papers during my tenth-grade boards.

My mind was whirling with the acronym A.L.L. and scrambling to find ways to deal with it.

The first major challenge was informing Ammi and Meher. Firoz and I decided to go at our own pace. 'It's just the beginning, so don't worry,' I told them, with all the phoney assurance I could muster. 'And it is fully curable.'

Yes, but how much would the therapy cost if it was treatable? My mind was racing with concerns. My three-year career at the Marriott had saved me what I believed was a reasonable sum. Thankfully, I had learned the art of saving early in life.

'Can I go to work while the treatment is going on?' I asked Dr Bhave.

'Since it is a cancer of white blood cells, chemotherapy will kill both healthy and cancerous cells. The blood cell count will plummet rapidly. This raises the likelihood of infection. If you become infected, we will have to discontinue treatment and focus on treating the infection. It is the risk of infection that will keep you from going to work,' the doctor gently stated.

I remembered how as kids my friends and I wouldn't have the money to buy kites. We were, however, desperate to fly one. If the borrow-now-repay-later plan succeeded, good for us. If that didn't work, running behind kites whose threads were cut and hauling them down from the trees did. Then there were the cricket matches where they collected 50 paise from each player. The ultimate prize of Rs 3 or Rs 5 would be awarded to the winner. There were also annual contests where they could win fantastic grand prizes of Rs 25 or Rs 50 (about 50 cents), which was an enormous boost for us kids.

That juggling of money had previously served me well. But now I found that my money would be wiped out during my first round of chemotherapy itself. Dr Bhave had estimated the cost at Rs 7 lakh (about $8500). Leukaemia patients are more susceptible to infection than others, which would add an additional 3–4 lakh rupees ($3600–$4800) to the bills. Furthermore, the full therapy would last around a year, followed by two years of maintenance.

I realised I was in for a few years. How was I going to arrange the money?

The Hunt for a Doctor

Another question nagged me. How do I find the best doctor fast before cancer spreads rapidly and kills me? Dr Bhave, the ever-helpful human being, recommended a few of his colleagues. Friends, colleagues and Marriott members provided further references.

Could he also find another hospital that was less expensive than Lilavati? I asked Dr Bhave for seven days to complete my R&D. What a week of going backwards and forwards it was!

First stop: Tata Memorial Hospital. The expenses were slightly lower, averaging Rs 5 lakh (about $6000) as opposed to Rs 7 lakh ($8500) at Lilavati. However, there was a lengthy wait. I would probably not be allowed to begin treatment very soon, despite having been referred by the head of Marriott's human resource team, having all my reports, and being a proven case of A.L.L.

Cross.

Second stop: Bombay Hospital, but the doctor wasn't available. I was asked to return later. Second round, the doctor was still not on the radar.

Cross.

The hospital run was getting to me, and I developed a high-grade fever. I called Dr Bhave at 7 p.m. The doctor answered his phone and suggested a line of treatment.

Third stop: Jaslok Hospital and Research Centre. Jaslok's protocols were almost the same as Lilavati's. So were the costs. Why travel so far then?

Cross.

Fourth stop: A series of haematologists, some referenced from Dr Bhave, others from friends and colleagues. At each clinic, I was introduced to the doctor's team. 'The doctor will see you once a week. Everything else is handled by his team,' was the common refrain.

Cross.

It was almost the end of the week, and another fever was peaking. This time I was shivering and feeling bitterly cold. It was 10 p.m. Is it too late to call Dr Bhave yet again? I tried anyway. Again, I got my answer and my medication.

This week-long research has been a waste of time and effort, I thought, as I huddled under my blanket. It dawned on me that my search for the best doctor was right here. At Lilavati. Which senior specialist answers his calls at any time of the night? And which senior specialist is so gracious as to answer and treat a person who is openly searching for other doctors and who may or may not end up being his patient? Dr Bhave is truly unique, I told myself. I was confident that if I must fight this disease, I need his confidence to help me. I need to trust him.

My rational mind advised me to speak to someone who has had a similar experience. But there were no blood cancer survivors whom he or anyone around him, doctors included, knew or were willing to disclose the names of. I needed to gauge the condition of my athletic body after three years of treatment. Why was cancer such a secret? Did people look like ghosts and so hid in their closets? I decided I would recover and become the brand ambassador of leukaemia.

As for Lilavati's expense, well, it was marginally higher. But, as Dr Bhave had mentioned, the chemotherapy would lead to a dip in white cell count, increasing the chances of infections. A super-hygienic facility like Lilavati would reduce the chances of infection and better my chances of survival.

I took the call and decided to entrust my life to Dr Bhave's hands. 'I know it's treatable and I'm going to get treated.'

3

WHEN ANGELS CAME KNOCKING

The final piece of the jigsaw was missing—the funds. I needed to kick off my cancer treatment pronto, but how was I going to do it? Nevertheless, I was determined to flush the cancer out of my system.

As a young boy, I was considered obstinate since I used to call my big brother by his name instead of 'bhai'. It peeved my father. My mother went back to sleep after filling containers with water from the community tap at 3.30 a.m. Naturally, our neighbours too woke up at the same time to fill their utensils with water. After this exercise in the middle of the night, everyone tried to get some sleep. I used to wake up at 4.30 to go for my runs, and the commotion annoyed my neighbours. When I was 10 or 12, I wanted to play more than attend school. It was the liberty to get up early and run. The testosterone was high, and we were young blokes with newfound freedom.

I would set off with a sprinkle of water, a handful of dates, and a couple of biscuits. On sunny days, I yearned for the dew on my skin, a brief respite from my packed house's heat. Even during cool December mornings, I didn't mind the effort to leave my cosy blanket or the freezing wind's slap when I stepped outside. The howls of the stray dogs didn't bother me either.

I would start ringing doorbells, or worse, banging on each of my mate's doors. The Shekhar and Sheetal brothers, who lived across the road, were first on my list. Rajesh resided next to them and then came my best friend Vinod, who was athletic as a stallion. Next in line was Niranjan, aka 'Annu', followed by Sridhar. Even the younger ones weren't exempt from my early wake-up calls. The doors of Swapnil, Kate and Vicky weren't spared either.

Some would grumble, growl, or hurl abuses at me, warning me never to come back. But that didn't bother me. I'd keep on knocking, and most of my friends would come running. We alternated between the Saki Naka-Powai Garden route and the airport, a good six to seven kilometres. We'd play either football or cricket during the holidays, and weekends were no excuse to sleep in. Mahaveer Nivas would battle it out against Chikiwala or Hassan Chawl in inter-chawl matches, all for the fantastic cash prize.

Back to the present, I had to rekindle my nerve and my devil-may-care attitude to finance my cancer treatment. I had to recapture the same mental freedom I had as a young lad. If I could knock then, I could knock now.

Blessings Amidst the Gloom

Life has a funny way of working things out. It builds us up, tests us, and when we least expect it, showers us with blessings. That's exactly what happened to me when I found out I had cancer.

I had no idea what was in store for me when I decided to knock on life's door, but it turns out that doors that I didn't even know existed were waiting to be opened. For example, I discovered that I had Rs 3 lakh ($3650) in medical insurance through the JW Marriott Relief Fund, which was a huge relief. The only dampener was that only Rs 50,000 (about $600) was available for cancer treatment, but that would take care of the initial procedures.

I realised that I needed to refocus and start informing my clients about my situation. Marriott's members had become like friends to me over the last three years, and I wanted to make sure I found someone to take care of them before I left for my treatment.

As I was going through my routine, a regular Marriott patron named Sadanand Shetty walked in. I felt like I had to tell him about my situation, so I did. To my surprise, he hugged me and offered to help. He said that commuting from Andheri to Lilavati was too far and that I risked infection, so he and an estate broker selected a few one-bedroom apartments near Lilavati for me to choose from. He even offered to take care of the deposit and rent for the duration of my treatment. I was in shock and couldn't find the words to thank him properly.

But Sadanand wasn't the only angel in my life. Shamshu Lalani, director of Lalani Group, offered me a one-bedroom apartment near Otter's Club, which was extremely close to Lilavati. He said he would get it cleaned up and painted for me, free of charge.

The outpouring of kindness did not stop there. Gautam Jasra (director, Jasra Graphics), Pankaj Razdan (then vice-president, ICICI Prudential), and Jaspal Singh Chandhok (owner, Balu India Crankshaft) all pitched in with funding for my treatment, and one of the Marriott members even called the Lilavati board of members to make sure I was taken care of.

I couldn't believe how lucky I was to have so many people looking out for me. Life had been a roller-coaster, but I felt grateful for the blessings that were showered on me when I needed them the most.

The Comrades

Leukaemia or not, I was determined to conquer The Comrades—the 90-mile annual ultra-marathon from Durban to Pietermaritzburg in South Africa. It was November 2004 and I set my sights on competing in 2006.

I felt proud of myself for embracing the right attitude to overcome all odds. The Comrades Marathon embodies my spirit—camaraderie, dedication, selflessness, perseverance, and ubuntu—everything I believe in.

Since 1921, three lakh runners had completed the race. I was convinced that I could be one of them. What attracted me to the marathon was its touchingly historic significance. It was established in honour of the South African World War I soldiers killed during the war. War veteran Vic Clapham, who founded the marathon, had trekked 2,700 kilometres through the sweltering heat of Africa. He had designed the marathon as a test of physical endurance, 'to celebrate mankind's spirit over adversity'.

Maybe that was life's way of telling me to run this historic race after conquering cancer. And I was sure I could. I had already triumphed over my humble chawl childhood, so why not this new adversity? I was determined to celebrate my spirit and overcome all odds.

PART II

Do not judge me by my success, judge me by how many times I fell down and got back up again.

—Nelson Mandela

4

THE PREP AND THE MOVE

On 19 November 2004, the first chemotherapy was scheduled, and I had to relocate to a temporary home in a week. With most of the funds collected and the packing underway, the fight for survival was picking up pace.

As I stepped out of the JW Marriott on my last working day before my medical break, Juhu was alive with twinkling lights. The following day, I was due at Lilavati Hospital, and I was eager to regain my health and take control of my life again.

My mother insisted I finish shifting my belongings before getting admitted, but I refused. Firoz was already stretched thin working at Reliance Industries in Airoli and helping with the packing at night. Against the hospital's protocol, I managed to convince Dr Bhave to allow me to be admitted alone.

While chemotherapy typically requires a full-time attendant due to the resultant weakness, nausea, and pain, there was no one else available to help me. Despite initial reluctance, Dr Bhave convinced the hospital management to allow me to manage my own treatment, including filling out forms, making payments, and getting discharged when the time came.

This newfound independence fuelled me with strength. My early morning runs had transformed into the biggest race of my life, and I was determined to emerge victorious.

Leaving Home, Starting Anew

My cancer wasn't my main concern—it was my mother's distress that troubled me the most. She was a mess, constantly hugging me and weeping. Two of her elder sisters had succumbed to cancer, and I felt sorry that she had to endure this again. As I packed my bags, my emotions ran high.

Dr Bhave informed me that the first chemotherapy cycle would require at least seven to fifteen days of hospitalisation. I saw this as an opportunity to catch up on my reading, a habit I had developed when I was working at Marriott. Initially, I started with books on nutrition and fitness, but I progressed to business books as well. I usually read on my two-and-a-half-hour commute by local train to work from Kalyan to Juhu. For the hospital, I packed my suitcase with clothes, masks, gadgets, and books. However, my mother took it as a sign that I would never return, and her tears started flowing again.

My apartment was cluttered with brown-paper cartons, suitcases and bundles, but it was the gloom in the air that weighed me down. Lilavati Hospital required me to check in at the reception desk before 8 a.m. As I hugged my mother and walked out, I took a deep breath and felt a strange sense of relief.

The crisp morning air filled me with hope as I rode in the autorickshaw from my Andheri home to Lilavati Hospital in Bandra. It felt like I was journeying through a tunnel, leaving behind one life for another. My mind buzzed with anticipation, but fear was absent. I was at peace, ready to embrace the unknown world of chemotherapy and hospitals.

Yet, guilt crept in, overpowering me. I felt sorry for putting Ammi through this illness at a time when she needed me the most. But I found solace in knowing that Firoz would assist at home and coordinate with Marriott's members for funding.

As I opened the protocol sheet, my heart raced. Words like radiation therapy, gamma rays and cytotoxic chemotherapy were daunting. I visualised toxic rays penetrating my skull, turning my blood into neon green and squid blue. I feared that my bones would dissolve and my body would melt away. I already felt soft and squishy like a jellyfish.

The word 'dexamethasone' caught my eye. As a professional nutritionist and fitness consultant certified by The American College of Sports Medicine, I knew it was a steroid that caused hunger and weight gain. Would I transform into a red-green Hulk?

As the autorickshaw jolted over a pothole, my thoughts wandered to the chemotherapy patients I had seen at Lilavati the previous week. All of them were bald. I accepted that side-effect but wondered if it was the only change I would experience.

Just a month ago, I was fit and toned with less than seven per cent fat in my body and was described as an 'athlete' in my medical records. Now, Dr Bhave's admission letter read, 'Shiraz Siddiqui, acute lymphoblastic leukaemia. Type: pre-B.'

Finally, the autorickshaw pulled up to the gates of Lilavati. The smell of hospitalisation hit me, and I glimpsed an arrow pointing to the morgue, which made me feel uneasy. But my spirit urged me on and I stepped inside. 'Get on with it, Shiraz,' I told myself, ready to face whatever lay ahead.

5

THE HOSPITAL SOJOURN BEGINS

Day 1, 8 a.m. As I approached Lilavati Hospital, the security guard eyed me sceptically and insisted on a baggage check. My large suitcase contained masks, medication, clothes, an iPad and a stack of books, which seemed to raise the guard's suspicion. I explained that I was advised to stay in the hospital for seven to fourteen days and I liked to read. After some friendly banter, he let me through.

Unexpectedly, the fragrance of incense hit me as I entered the lobby. On my right, there was a small temple, and on my left was the reception desk. I handed over my admission letter and the forms I had filled out earlier. The receptionist looked at me quizzically and asked, 'Who is the patient?' to which I replied, 'I am'. I had to explain my situation yet again before receiving the necessary forms.

I then headed to the accounts department to deposit Rs 25,000 ($300) and collect my receipt and visitors' passes. Afterwards, I took the elevator to the chemotherapy ward on the eighth floor. I could have taken the stairs, but I wanted to take my time and soak up the ambience.

At the nursing desk, the head nurse greeted me with a warm smile. She asked who would be attending to me, and I replied, 'Myself. I will be alone.' The smile vanished from her face, and I had to narrate my story yet again. She called Dr Bhave to confirm my situation. Once she received confirmation, she asked a nurse to escort me to my room.

I couldn't afford a deluxe room, so I opted for a twin-sharing room, which came with a caveat. If my white blood cell counts dropped, I would have to move to a single room due to a higher risk of infection. Luckily, my bed faced the window, and the view from it made the hospital feel like a hotel.

Gradually, I adjusted to the brightness of the white light in my room, noticing that my shoes and clothes had been locked away as per Lilavati's complete ban on anything from home to protect chemotherapy patients from catching infections. I changed into a blue uniform with tiny checks, pyjamas and a shirt with ties on the sides. Alone in my room, I watched the busy street outside and killed time. From my window, I could see the main road opposite, the lanes that bifurcated from it, and the Maharashtra Education Trust's (M.E.T) campus below. I even spotted a pizzeria that was once part of my life. But now, this bed, the astringent smell of sanitiser, and the blue clothes were my reality.

The next morning, breakfast comprised cornflakes, milk and idlis. The staff came and went, medicating, changing bedsheets and attending to other tasks. Dr Bhave walked in, extending his usual friendly good mornings, and informed me of the day's agenda, which included hydration, a blood test, some tablets and, finally, the drugs.

Before we got started, the doctor introduced me to the entire staff on the floor, especially the nursing staff. By the time I returned to my window-facing bed, my bag with the saline solution was ready and I had to lie still for three hours. A completely tasteless Indian meal arrived for lunch, which I chewed through like a model patient. I was administered some antacids and anti-nausea drugs, followed by soda-mint tablets, which helped maintain the body's pH balance.

Soon tea and biscuits arrived, followed by the first chemotherapy drug, which was administered intravenously. Contrary to my expectations, it was easy-peasy with no adverse reactions. And just like that, Day 1 was over.

Little did I know that my day had only just begun. As the evening drew in, my stomach began to bloat and hyper-acidic unease set in. My body started to react to the day's toxic chemical intake.

But my mind was briefly distracted when two members of Marriott walked in for a surprise visit. Despite the pain, I put on a smile. They joked and offered words of encouragement. 'If you have to get cancer, this is the best type,' they said, and their warmth strengthened me.

When dinner arrived, I tried to force-feed myself for the first time in my life, but to no avail. After a while, I called a nurse and requested some anti-nausea drugs. I had to wait for an extremely uncomfortable hour before the drugs took effect. Finally, I managed to down a single *paratha* and call it a night.

Sleep was elusive. The discomfort and new surroundings made it difficult. My roommate, an elderly woman suffering from a relapse, was also in pain. Her son, a doctor, couldn't do much to relieve her suffering. No one felt like turning on the small television to distract us.

My eyes closed, but my mind kept ticking.

* * *

Day 2, 7.45 a.m. onwards. The kind-hearted nurses skilfully extracted more blood, carefully collecting samples for pathology tests in preparation for the upcoming round of chemotherapy. Their expertise and precision were reassuring amidst the anticipation of what lay ahead.

'Monitor your urine,' a nurse gently reminded me, her voice laced with concern. 'It's absolutely vital to keep a close eye on your water intake and output during chemotherapy. Kidney function loss stands as one of the prominent side effects of this treatment.'

An hour later, the momentous session of chemotherapy commenced. Nausea intensified with a relentless force. Even the prescribed anti-nausea medication proved ineffective in alleviating this tormenting sensation. The unsettling realisation that constant vomiting could lead to weight loss gnawed at my mind, fuelling a growing sense of worry. Losing weight would not only weaken my body but could potentially hinder my ability to receive the vital chemotherapy I so desperately needed.

6

GETTING BACK CONTROL

As a nutritionist, I decided to take matters into my hands and reached out to Lilavati's dietician. I requested a food management plan with a minimum of 1,600 calories a day, filled with nutrient-dense food, every two to three hours—even if I could not manage to reach the required 2,000 calories per day target.

She introduced me to the chef who promised to fulfil any order, any time of the day. I requested small, nutrient-dense meals every two to three hours with no empty calories but high in energy.

I felt I was back in control.

The nausea worsened, causing bloating and severe stomach cramps, indicating my body's negative reaction to the foreign chemotherapy drugs.

'If I'm going to beat this disease, I need to manage the side effects—physically and mentally. And what better way to do that than by doing what I love most: sports. My mind and body need at least an hour of exercise every day,' I resolved to myself. I created a timetable that juggled doctors' schedules, chemotherapy timings, pathology test timings, C.T. scans, X-rays and 2-D echo timings to fit in exercise every day.

I planned a morning routine of breathing exercises and meditation, followed by light exercises to build physical and mental strength. I made a list of all the foods with energy, high-density of nutrients, vitamins and antioxidants. Adequate rest was a top priority; seven to eight hours of sleep was mandatory to recover from chemotherapy.

On the second night, my body was reacting worse than anticipated. Dark thoughts crept in, but I refused to let cancer win. 'If I can plan this successfully, I will make it through one of the toughest periods of my life. Failure to plan is planning for failure. I won't let that happen,' I promised myself.

'Focus,' I repeated to myself, determined to overcome my natural inclination to avoid the hospital. The thought of being confined to a sterile room was unbearable.

But then, my spirit intervened and reminded me, 'Remember when you focused on studying for your S.S.C Board exams, despite your aversion to academics?'

That was true. Throughout my schooling at St Anthony's High School in Saki Naka, I was more interested in sports than academics. I often skipped lectures to play for a few extra minutes, and opened my books only fifteen days before the exams—unless there were district or state-level games scheduled in between.

In class nine, the red marks on my calendar were too frequent for my parents to ignore. But it was the prelims in class X that proved disastrous—I failed in four subjects. My parents were furious. I was worried about my future.

So I made a decision. For the next three months, I attended every class and studied hard, cramming as much as possible. And it paid off—I secured 55 per cent in my Board exams, a milestone that my family celebrated with Pradhan's laddoos distributed throughout the chawl! For the first time in ten years of schooling, I focused on my studies and achieved this milestone.

Now, faced with a life-threatening illness, I needed that same level of focus.

On Day 3, I took control despite my health issues. I woke up before the nurse and headed to the nurse's station with my saline bottle. 'May I have the list of chemotherapy drugs I am being given?' I asked. As a nutritionist and fitness consultant, I needed to understand the chemicals being injected into my body to manage my nausea, acidity and joint pain through nutrition and exercise, I told her.

The senior nurse was intrigued, a trifle hesitant, but eventually relented and sent me the list. I then requested some basic books to further my understanding of the subject. With the arrival of the books, I added two hours of research to my daily routine, along with breathing exercises and meditation in the mornings and nutrient-dense meals.

Within hours, word spread around Lilavati Hospital that I was a professional nutritionist and fitness consultant and, soon, even doctors came to analyse my knowledge! Helping others in this way kept my mind engaged and made me feel that I was back on the job, albeit in a different way.

* * *

As the first week at Lilavati passed, I grew accustomed to the rhythms of hospitalisation, and my timetable seemed to be working well. As I breathed in the Friday morning sun, I had only one procedure left before discharge: experiencing 'the L.P.' or lumbar puncture.

The staff was bustling around. Needles and syringes of various sizes and sample bottles were arranged on a trolley beside my bed. A mask was placed over my face, and Dr Bhave arrived to explain the procedure. 'We will enter between L4 and L5 to take a sample of the cerebral spinal fluid and then inject a chemotherapy drug. This area and the brain are the hiding spot for a mass of cancer cells.'

After sanitising my back, local anaesthesia was injected. The doctor waited, again feeling my back to check if it was safe to start the procedure. I felt the needle enter my spine and though there was no pain, a strange tingling sensation made me start sweating profusely. Long minutes ticked by in silence.

'Please cough,' instructed a nurse, and a sample was collected. 'Now, we just have to inject the chemotherapy and you will be done,' assured Dr Bhave. The syringe was filled and the injection was administered.

'It's done,' said Dr Bhave, patting my shoulder, 'Just lie low and don't take a bath for 24 hours.' I was instructed to lie on my back and then on my stomach for a total of five hours.

As discomfort and pain rose with every passing minute, I muttered to myself, 'Just four more hours.'

7

OUT INTO THE WORLD AGAIN

After fifteen days of confinement and constant medical attention, I was finally back in the world. Everything had changed. My new home was in Bandra, so no more long travels. As I stepped inside, the scent of fresh paint welcomed me. Ammi had done wonders with the place. But my elation quickly turned into caution when I noticed the open windows.

'We need mosquito nets on all the windows immediately,' I told Ammi.

'Take a breath, Sheru,' she replied, beaming with joy to have me back. It was a relief to see her smile again.

But first things first. I called the local carpenter to install the mosquito nets as soon as possible. Fortunately, fumigation and pest control had already been taken care of. The complete blood count (CBC) I had taken before leaving the hospital had left me anxious. My white blood cell count was already low, hovering around 4,200, and under the impact of continued oral chemotherapy, it was expected to dip even further over the next ten days. Dr Bhave had warned me about the risk of infection.

I pushed my worries aside and savoured the joy of being back home with my mother.

'You've lost so much weight,' she said.

'Mothers are always like that,' I teased her. But I knew I was three kilos lighter. 'Well, I'm here now, so you can feed me as much as possible. No dietary restrictions for me,' I said grinning.

Raw food was off-limits because they could cause gut infections. It was Ammi's homemade meals for now.

The next day, as I combed my hair, it started falling out in clumps. I ran my hand along my scalp, and more hair came out. It had only been a day since I returned home, and I could already feel the chemotherapy's side effects. I decided to go bald and called my barber home, first ensuring that he didn't have any cold or cough symptoms.

Over the next few days, I realised that life had completely changed. Dr Bhave's warning about 'lifestyle changes' made sense now. No one with even a minor cold, cough, or infection could visit me. Ammi had to manage her health and keep everything hygienic, from meals to bedding.

But the biggest change was that I couldn't step out. However, I found joy in watching Ammi go for her daily walks to Carter Road. She came back beaming with happiness. My only outings were to Lilavati Hospital and back every two to three days for blood tests. Who would have thought that putting on a mask and hopping into an autorickshaw for a hospital visit would feel like a joyride? I felt like a prisoner who relished every moment of freedom.

* * *

Preparing for Chemotherapy: A Crisp Diet Plan

After a brief respite, I was ready for my second round of chemotherapy. My immune system was weak, and I was on antibiotics to combat minor infections. Along with this, I was taking chemotherapy drugs to control uric acid levels and specific supplements to maintain haemoglobin levels. It was crucial to plan my diet accordingly.

To begin with, I added jaggery to my morning and afternoon tea, a rich source of iron. Then, I started making granola at home with jaggery and cooked figs. To add more nutrients, I included cooked fruits like bananas, custard apples and apples in my diet. Although my palate had developed a constant metallic taste, I experimented with different recipes, like adding roasted almonds and nuts to my porridge or blending a milkshake with cow's milk, almond milk and fruits. This dietary change stayed with me throughout my illness and beyond.

Due to the chemotherapy drugs, my appetite had decreased, and I often experienced nausea, hyperacidity and bloating. Therefore, I prioritised nutritionally superior, calorie-rich and energy-boosting foods. My mother and I enjoyed experimenting with the diet plan and even sautéed our salads.

Throughout my illness, I continued to research and educate myself on nutrition and enrolled in a course on the toxic effects of chemicals and pesticides.

Despite the challenges, I felt empowered by taking control of my diet and making conscious choices to support my health.

* * *

The Second Round of Chemotherapy

Returning to Lilavati for my second round of chemotherapy wasn't as daunting this time. After two weeks of being home, the ups and downs of life seemed to have become easier to handle. As I made my way to the hospital, I couldn't help but reflect on how quickly the mind adapts to life's challenges.

Just a few weeks ago, my first rickshaw ride from my Andheri home to Lilavati was filled with anxiety. Now, it almost felt like just another commute to work.

Dr Bhave had recommended the German protocol, which involved several minor and major chemotherapies. This time, the treatment began with a lumbar puncture. Despite being warned about the post-lumbar puncture syndrome, I had not experienced it before. This time, however, it hit me with a vengeance in the form of a severe headache.

Lilavati allowed me to return home after five days, but the headache persisted. I tried everything to ease the throbbing pain—from placing my head on a pillow to resting it on a windowsill or a wall. But the pain was so severe that I had to maintain a head low position to avoid feeling dizzy.

As I endured the pain, my mind drifted back to another challenge I had faced as a child. I remembered how, as the baby of the family, I used to play football with boys seven years older than me. I had just started swimming lessons with them when one of them pushed me into the deep end of the pool. The memory of that moment and the exchange of a few colourful words spurred my determination to master swimming.

With only Rs 50 as pocket money for the entire summer vacation, I couldn't afford to spend it all on bus fare on the ride to the pool. So, I ran instead. My friend, Ishwar, had promised to coach me, but he only came along for a day. Undeterred, I watched and learned, and within two weeks, I was able to swim the entire length of the pool on my own.

Now, as I battled the post-lumbar puncture syndrome, I remembered how I had overcome my fear of drowning and had become a champion swimmer. Like back then, I was determined to overcome this challenge too. Both experiences taught me the power of determination in the face of seemingly overwhelming obstacles.

8

BACK IN HOSPITAL

It had been almost three weeks since the lumbar procedure, and I could no longer bear the headaches. The post-lumbar puncture syndrome had lasted longer than I had anticipated. I rushed to the Outpatient Department (OPD) at Lilavati to see Dr Bhave, but he was late and there was a long queue of patients waiting to see him. The headache was making me dizzy, and my eyes were watering profusely. People around me thought I was sobbing and tried to console me. I lay my head down on a chair, breathless, telling myself to hold on.

Finally, when Dr Bhave saw me, he discovered that my haemoglobin count had dropped to as low as six! He instructed me to get admitted to Lilavati immediately. 'If you know people who can donate blood, please call them. It will lower the cost of transfusion,' he advised.

Without much hope, I called the Marriott Fitness Centre. However, to my surprise, many groups of people turned up willing to donate blood for me. Throughout the week, people kept trickling in to donate blood. My entire department, and even departments like laundry, housekeeping and human resources, came forward to donate blood!

Around 64 people turned up for the five bottles of blood I needed, and the rest was banked for later use. The hospital staff pointed out to me that it was a unique display of solidarity that Lilavati had rarely seen.

As I lay low, waiting for the headache to subside, I told myself, 'Miracles never cease. I had angels and I didn't even know it.'

* * *

Amidst physical pain, confusion and sensitivity to the surroundings, the cancer ward was not the happiest of places. But one patient, a chirpy lady with colon cancer, taught me a valuable lesson. She was blissfully unaware of her aggressive cancer and happy to be recovering. Her son, an anaesthesiologist, confided in me that she might not survive for more than six months. Her positivity left me wondering why I couldn't be the same.

Just when my treatment was facing challenges, my body reacted wildly to a viral infection after receiving foreign blood. With my temperature touching 105°C, I lay shivering and stressing about what was going to happen. Dr Bhave was called in at around 1.30 a.m., and he decided to move me to the isolation ward as my white blood cell count had dropped to below 1,500.

Alone in the isolation ward that night, I told myself to gather courage and stay positive. I trusted Dr Bhave's line of treatment and waited for the fever to subside. For the first time, I wished for a hand to hold.

* * *

Life In a Box

Day 1: Since most of the rooms at Lilavati were occupied, my previous twin-sharing room was stripped and transformed into a strict isolation ward as per Dr Bhave's orders. This was my box: a small single room available with no space to move about. It had a tiny window overlooking the other building of the hospital. Only doctors and nurses were allowed in, after sanitising their hands, wearing masks and gloves, and removing their footwear. It was my first complete isolation experience.

Day 2: The fever persisted and Dr Bhave called in a specialist who ordered more tests. The reports would come in 48 hours.

Day 3: It became a waiting game. I was alone with my thoughts, haunted by the warnings in the books about the fatal complications of infections when the body's immunity was low. During times like these, ignorance is bliss, I told myself.

Day 4: There was relief as the reports showed no serious infections, only a viral fever. But my low white blood cell count rendered my immunity unable to fight it.

Day 5: I remained isolated, with only Dr Bhave and a nurse checking my vital stats. My mind refused to quieten. I felt trapped.

Day 6: It brought positive signs as my temperature dropped, but my spirit oscillated between optimism and depression. Managing my mind was becoming a significant challenge.

Day 7: Dr Bhave's previous advice on lifestyle changes took on a new meaning. Somehow, I had to quieten my mind, and I felt like a failure for the first time. Tears rolled down and I didn't even realise I was crying.

Day 8: It was filled with uncertainty about my future and my ability to face the outside world. The four walls seemed to encase my mind too. I had no clue how many more days I would have to be in this box. Is this what Nelson Mandela faced when he was imprisoned for so many years? I felt trapped.

Day 9: The fever subsided and my white blood cell count rose, but my ESR counts were too high, indicating inflammation within the body. I expressed my frustration to Dr Bhave who gently advised me to be patient for another 24 hours.

Day 10: It dragged on as I waited to be discharged. When Dr Bhave finally gave me the green light, I was ready to face the worst, thanks to my ten days of isolation. I felt nothing could be worse than this experience.

* * *

I Have to Get Through This!

'I can do this,' I thought, determined to push through the aftermath of chemotherapy. 'The maintenance treatment' awaited me, two years of minor chemotherapy cycles once a month followed by five days of steroids. The intrathecal or lumbar puncture was necessary once every quarter. But by August 2005, my main chemotherapy protocols had concluded, and I was able to rejoin Marriott. Despite not being as fit as before, it was a glorious feeling to be back at work.

Chemotherapy drugs tend to bloat you, and I was no exception. My weight had reached 92 kilos, and the steroids made me insatiably hungry. The cravings were so intense that I always felt desperate for food. My sugar levels shot up to 200, way beyond the normal range of 110. Managing my diet and taking insulin shots became mandatory. I grudgingly accepted this dependence on medication, often chuckling to myself as I called myself the 'unfit fitness coach'.

The steroids also had a debilitating effect on me, making me weak and robbing me of muscle mass, especially in my legs. I could not even sustain small tasks. Insomnia caused by the steroids made me toss and turn till 3 a.m. each night.

Despite that, I began my mornings early, practising Tai Chi breathing for 10 to 15 minutes. I could only manage light, low-impact cardio and cycling for ten minutes at low intensity. Stretching became my go-to exercise to free up my stiff muscles, and my workout routine aimed for 45 minutes, which would burn around 200 calories. It was just not enough to produce results, given my food intake.

In February 2006, I was prescribed statins, a cholesterol-lowering medication, as my levels had increased. However, I could not raise my workout intensity without getting cramps, dehydration and feeling unwell. My eagerness to get off cholesterol and sugar medication made me repeat the same mistake thrice, resulting in back spasms and severe hamstring cramps.

'I must respect my body's limitations and work within my capabilities,' I reminded myself.

From August 2005 to July 2007, the drugs and routine hospital visits continued, causing me to slow down but never give up on my fitness journey. Finally, in August 2007, I received good news after a long time. Dr Bhave gave me a clean chit and announced that 'the maintenance phase is over. We will not require any more chemotherapy or steroids'. I was now cancer-free, free from all drugs and hospital visits. I had finally conquered!

9

LIFE IN 21-DAY CYCLES

Two years of fluctuating fitness levels during maintenance therapy felt like an eternity to me. Immaturely, I thought I would be done with cancer in a year. However, it took three years—2004 had become 2007. Now that it was over, I wanted to work hard on my diet. I aimed to wean myself off insulin injections and statins while controlling my hunger pangs. I decided to plan for 21 days at a time.

The First 21 days

Step 1: Do the Obvious

First, I calculated my calories versus my Basal Metabolic Rate (BMR) and current activity levels. With a BMR of 1,600, my current activity was burning only 1,000 calories a day. Plus, I was consuming a whopping 3,500 calories! The plan was to add an extra 40 minutes of early morning walking and taper down the calories gradually, starting with a 10 per cent reduction. I cut out hidden calories from sodium and sugar from indirect sources such as biscuits. I maintained this plan for 21 days and could see the results.

Step 2: Eat Clean

I included 200 metres of slow jogging for the first time, but my heart rate shot up to 180 beats per minute (bpm); the normal range is 60–100 bpm. I switched to 'interval training', which comprised 200 metres of exceedingly slow jogging bordering on 'almost shuffling' followed by a recovery walk of 600 metres. This way I would try to cover at least 3 to 3.5 kilometres per day.

I tapered the calories in my diet by another 10 per cent and shifted my focus from just calories to 'eating clean'. It doesn't matter if you are a vegetarian or even vegan. If you do not find food which is clean and free of pesticides, it's not going to help. It's a slow poison that could lead to infections and even cancer. I scanned for produce which was free of antibiotics. I looked for farmers' markets in the city and searched for as much organic produce as I could get.

The next step was to eliminate refined flour and refined sugar. I eliminated bread and replaced it with homemade rotis, either wheat or preferably millets or ragi. I was still not allowed to eat raw food, but I added more cooked fruits to my diet.

Step 3: Say No to Refined

I avoided refined products and packaged foods. Again, I could see clear results.

Step 4: Reduce Carbohydrates

I reduced all carbohydrates by 10 per cent and switched to moderate or low glycaemic index foods. I changed from white rice to brown rice, or mostly no rice at all. If I craved a khichdi, I made it more out of green mung dal and kept the rice minimal. I limited my sugar intake to fruits, the occasional date or two, or some honey.

Step 5: Further Reduction

I further tapered my diet by 10 per cent, reaching 2,300 calories a day. That's still a lot, technically, but I was still seeing good results. My hunger pangs were under control, and I was feeling fresh. Most importantly, I was able to slow jog continuously for three kilometres, and my heart rate, which previously took at least four minutes to settle down, now calmed down in two minutes.

In three months, I saw remarkable results and achieved a big milestone in my life—getting off insulin completely!

Next Goal: Eliminate Statins

I was still taking 20 mg of statin each night. So, I repeated my lipid profile test and saw that it appeared normal. I asked my physician to reduce it further, and he agreed to have me take it every other night.

To regulate my cholesterol, I developed a plan. This included increasing the intake of green, leafy vegetables and enzymes in my diet. I began soaking mung, legumes and seeds each night, and steaming or boiling them for dinner with unprocessed apple cider vinegar. I made this a routine, just like taking my medication.

I also started doing more strength training to build up my leg muscles, aiming to run 10 kilometres and cycle

25 kilometres without stopping. I love setting goals because they help me focus and stay motivated.

Gradually, I increased my running to three times a week, cycling twice a week, and strength training twice a week, with one hour of stretching on a separate day.

On day 35, I met my target, running 10 kilometres and cycling 25 kilometres without stopping, followed by 30 minutes of strength training. The next day, I took another lipid profile test, and the results were incredibly motivating. The doctor suggested I stop taking statins until the next lipid profile test, and then restart by taking them twice a week for two weeks before stopping completely.

This meant another month of exercise and a proper diet, but the next lipid profile test showed that I was in great shape. I had returned to my pre-cancer weight of 75 kilos with 14 per cent fat, shedding the 92 kilos and 29 per cent fat from before. Insomnia, blood sugar issues and high cholesterol were gone. Most importantly, all my pathological parameters were normal for the first time since my leukaemia diagnosis.

I realised that setting goals for myself had been a significant help, and I congratulated myself for not making excuses. In February 2008, after eight months of hard work, I was happy to have my life and body back in shape. I was extremely proud of my achievement!

10

THE RELAPSE

I had no intention of slowing down my training and diet. Instead, I wanted to increase the intensity. But something felt off. A regular headache had been increasing for the past week, making me wonder if I was pushing myself too hard. Not wanting to take any chances, I consulted Dr Bhave again, who sent me to a neurologist. A scan revealed a clot in one of the veins in my brain, the reason behind the headaches.

The neurologist immediately prescribed medications and anticoagulant therapy. I had to monitor my blood viscosity levels carefully to maintain the delicate ratio between thick and thin blood. Regular check-ups and pathological tests resumed at the rate of twice a week, and I soon discovered that maintaining the fragile balance was no easy task. The drugs would interact with the food, necessitating fine-tuning of my diet. Even simple cold-cough syrups could hamper the efficacy of the new drugs.

This impacted my exercise regime as well. I had to be careful while performing high-intensity workouts, as my body took time to get used to the new drug. I learned to manage the dose and watch out for physical signs to prevent serious complications such as haemorrhage. Every Tuesday and

Friday, I returned for tests. There was this constant feeling that the medicines didn't want to leave me.

Despite this, I refused to let it stop me from training. Within a month, I was once again comfortable and ready to build intensity. 'I can handle any situation and just keep going,' I told Dr Bhave confidently. The year passed by, and the scans came out clear. The clot had completely disappeared, and I was allowed to stop the medication. It was almost 2009, and what a year it had been!

The Toy Train Called Life

To get my life back on track, I set two goals: rebuild my bank balance and buy a house within the next few years. Despite working at the Marriott for a couple of years, all my earnings went towards treatment, leaving me with zero savings. Determined to make a change, I started working longer hours, taking on more clients and doing more personal training and local consultations.

Meanwhile, Ammi broached the subject of me getting married. I told her I was fine with it and only hoped that the girl would understand my journey and me. That got Ammi looking for prospective brides! Photographs were regularly exchanged, and a few meetings were arranged. Finally, one alliance clicked. The girl's family was informed about the cancer and were comfortable with my health history.

'Don't rush into an early wedding date, Ammi,' I requested, 'let me just settle down a bit.' Both families agreed and everything was going as per plan.

Ready For Relapse

12 April 2009. Worried that my cancer had returned, I visited a gastroenterologist who diagnosed me with a minor infection and prescribed antibiotics and probiotics. However, my physical condition didn't improve, and my fears of a cancer relapse grew.

After a blood test revealed a further dip in haemoglobin, I contacted Dr Bhave. He instructed me to do pathology tests immediately and showed the same sense of urgency as before. A bone marrow biopsy confirmed my worst fears: *it was a relapse.*

In April 2009, exactly five years after my first cancer diagnosis, I found myself back in the same hospital room, undergoing the same procedure. This time, however, my frame of mind was completely different. Despite feeling invincible during my first battle with cancer, the truth was far from it.

Dr Bhave confirmed the relapse and instructed us to start chemotherapy urgently. He never minced his words. 'This time, we need to combine regular chemotherapy with a protocol known as R-chop, which includes a biological medication known as Rituximab,' he said, emphasising his words to gauge my reaction. I waited for the catch.

'A single shot of this injection costs around Rs 1.2 lakh ($1450). You'll need at least eight. The total protocol is estimated at around Rs 18 lakh (about $22,000),' he said, pausing for effect.

'And, Shiraz,' he added gently, 'it's time to start looking for a bone marrow transplant donor.'

I was in the present moment, unable to think beyond it. 'I have about Rs 7 lakh ($8,500) saved. I'll somehow manage the rest.'

'Let's get started with the treatment immediately,' he responded. For some reason, I was in a hurry this time. I didn't want to dwell on arranging the money, or the other alarming issues that come with hospitalisation, like stay, work and family.

It was 12 April 2009. I was admitted within the next two days.

* * *

I first shared the news with my brother, Firoz, who was working abroad. Then, I informed my clients and everyone at the Marriott. Lastly, I broke the news to Ammi, sugarcoating the truth and lying about the severity of the situation. Dr Bhave had warned that the relapse would be much more aggressive than before and outlined a treatment plan of at least eight months.

Ammi was sharp and cross-questioned me about why I needed to be admitted immediately. Despite being trained in self-control through Tai Chi, I grew annoyed and frustrated with her. I packed my bags decisively and left for the hospital the next day, leaving Ammi unconvinced. I knew she would call Firoz for more answers.

As I left, I hugged her tightly, knowing she would cry once I shut the door. My eyes were moist, and I put on sunglasses to hide my emotions. The day was 14 April 2009. Within twenty days, a 'minor stomach infection' had transformed into a major cancer relapse.

* * *

Returning to Lilavati was easier on the soul this time. The R-chop protocol was true to its word, and it took a toll on my body. Within two days of starting chemotherapy, my white cell count dropped to under 500. Dr Bhave ordered immediate isolation. Imprisonment was back. The costs were high, but I was mentally prepared this time. I knew I had to fight it, but my body had other plans. It challenged me more than I was prepared for, but I fought to regain control. After a few days in isolation, my white cell count rose enough for me to be discharged.

The prospective bride's family was informed about the relapse, and they were disarmingly sympathetic. 'It's okay,' they said. 'We can wait.'

'No, my son would like to cancel plans,' said Ammi softly, 'We don't know what life has in store for him. We don't want to ruin your girl's life.'

The second cycle of R-chop chemotherapy was scheduled for three weeks after the first, followed by ten days of isolation—my third stint. I watched the runners at Worli Sea Face from the isolation ward and longed to join them. Will I ever? 'Shut up,' said my spirit, admonishing me.

I managed to get out of the box and get discharged, but within five days, I was back in Lilavati with a viral infection. Again, I fought and went home, only to return to Lilavati within seven days with another viral infection. Yet again, I fought against it and went home.

11

A CANCER PATIENT CAN HAVE DREAMS TOO

'I'm living my life one chemotherapy cycle at a time. With all these cytotoxic chemicals, I never know which infection or breath could be my last,' I mused to myself. Death was becoming more real, but strangely fear was absent. I saw it as a discovery, a chance to explore a new path.

'In acceptance comes freedom from fear, right?' I wondered.

Fortunately, I went into remission just as the third cycle of chemotherapy began. My body responded well to the treatment, but I knew I wanted to do something more with my life. 'I don't want to die as an employee of a company. I want to become an entrepreneur,' I confided to Ammi one night.

She smiled, but I could sense her worries. It had been six years since Abu passed away, and Ammi had been through a lot. But I had a mission.

'I know Abbu failed as an entrepreneur, but I want to succeed where he failed. It's always been my dream,' I said, trying not to hurt her.

My parents had never stifled my dreams or pressured me into traditional professions. Even though sports was not considered a viable career choice, they supported me. 'Follow your passion, but do your duty too,' Ammi would say.

This time, she took it well. Relief made me sleep easier.

* * *

With renewed determination, I knew that pursuing my dreams was my priority. Explaining my plans to Ammi, I shared my vision for a wellness business that was focused on holistic health rather than just fitness. In my free moments, whether at the hospital or home, I spent my time wisely by reaching out to successful business owners. They became my tutors, and my clients turned into my teachers. I was constantly researching, reading, questioning and learning.

These past five years of battling cancer had given me profound insights. I had leaned on my doctors for advice on my cancer, the necessary nutrition and drug interactions with my body. I requested references for reading materials and explanations for what I didn't understand.

Now, I was pursuing my clients for their business acumen. Learning various business structures such as proprietorship, private limited and limited liability, I gained a deep understanding of the procedures of registration, logos, trademarks and websites. I developed knowledge about budgets and strategies for business.

In search of a company name, a Marriott member offered me a disc with corporate names, and Virtus appealed to me. In Latin, Vir means man, and the word stands for manliness, ambition and excellence. For me, it exuded energy and positivity, which inspired my logo—a plant that grows green and beautiful from roots to leaves, one step at a time.

Finally, I designed my first business card as an entrepreneur.

Shiraz Siddiqui
Founder & CEO
Virtus Wellness Private Limited

All that remained now was to fight and beat this disease.

Hiccups Again, but Focus Is on Business

Chemotherapy cycles four and five passed with the usual ups and downs. I persevered, focusing on my business. One day, there was unbearable pain in my ribs and I had difficulty breathing. I was rushed to the casualty at Lilavati and given antibiotics and life-saving drugs. The tests showed severe jaundice. I was forced into a twelve-day isolation, my fourth, followed by three agonising days of being kept under observation.

On day 16, I was finally discharged, but my immunity was compromised. My seventh chemotherapy round would commence only if my blood reports were normal in a week.

The question on my mind was, 'Will it ever end? Or will I?'

Welcome Entrepreneurship

I rapidly ascended the corporate ladder at Marriott, despite my absences due to my illness. My success made me the most sought-after trainer, and I was on the cusp of becoming the fitness director. However, I had different plans. I was eager to resign and pursue my dreams.

On 26 December 2009, I resigned from Marriott. The head of Human Resources called me for a meeting. When I handed my new CEO visiting card to him, he was puzzled and concerned as he had never heard of the brand. I explained that it was my company, and that I was the founder. He was happy to see my dream come true but concerned about me quitting while I was still recovering from my illness. I reassured him that I needed to live my dreams before it was too late. We parted on a firm handshake and I promised to consult the Marriott members and help them if needed. However, I had to serve a three-month notice period and was responsible for training my second-in-line to take over after me.

Meanwhile, I started my seventh round of chemotherapy, but despite the physical limitations, my mind was free and I spent all my time planning my company. The thrill of pursuing my dream made this the most exciting time of my life.

A few days later, Dr Jayant Gandhi from Shri Vile Parle Kelavani Mandal (S.V.K.M.), which had well-known colleges like Mithibai and Narsee Monjee Institute of Management Studies under its banner, expressed interest in starting a health and wellness programme for his students.

I was hopeful about being chosen after multiple interviews, and even other fitness industry veterans showed their support. Despite the ongoing chemotherapy and constant pain, my excitement was uncontainable and my smile never faded.

Virtus Is Born

With only two days left before my last day at Marriott, the place that made my childhood dreams come true, I couldn't help but wonder if I would have had the courage to quit if I hadn't got cancer. Life has its plans even if we don't see them.

On 20 April 2010, I established Virtus as a private limited company with the help of my friend and genealogist, Pranav Anam, who agreed to sit on the board as director. The very next day, I received a call congratulating me on winning the contract for the S.V.K.M. Trust. Dr Gandhi appreciated our well-defined, scientific protocol and focus on safety, and he trusted our client-handling skills as a service industry veteran. I was elated to have landed my first contract ever!

However, I needed to hire trainers quickly for the S.V.K.M. Trust gym programme, which hadn't started yet. I began hosting weekly nutrition classes for students, which turned out to be a great learning experience for both parties.

Soon after, the second contract came in from Dharmesh Jain, chairman and managing director of Nirmal Group. Jain had approached me for personalised training a year earlier, but my cancer relapse prevented us from moving forward. Now, he not only needed my services, but he also wanted me to take care of the health and fitness of Nirmal's employees.

As word spread that the Marriott trainer had started his own company, my former colleagues joined Virtus too. Nitin Rane, an expert long-distance swimmer and a friend from Marriott, moved with me and was soon joined by Rakesh Ghanekar, one of my assistants.

Virtus couldn't afford their Marriott salaries, but they believed in me and my company. Little did we know that their decision to join Virtus' leadership team would transform their lives.

I hired Nilesh Padlekar as our first personal trainer, referred by Rane. Virtus then secured its third contract to manage the corporate gym for Windsor Realty. I was grateful for the good start, as within three months of launching Virtus Wellness, we had one educational institute, two corporate companies, and a personalised trainee under our banner. With a team of eight trainers, I promised them that it was just the beginning.

* * *

As I worked on the jigsaw puzzle, I couldn't help but feel happy. It was enjoyable to solve, just like building my business. My friend and now a director at Virtus, Pranav, generously shared his office space and administrative staff with me. With his guidance, I found a chartered accountant to manage Virtus's books.

Despite the constant pain, I felt like the happiest person on Earth. I was fulfilling my family's dream and becoming an entrepreneur. I wanted to establish a personal training business that catered to high-net-worth individuals and founders of companies who needed personalised nutrition and residential training services.

To attract clients, I reached out to my network, including Dharmesh Jain and other Marriott members for references. Soon, the Nirmal family, including Mahek Jain, his daughter, became our clients. Nilesh handled Virtus's strength and conditioning sessions, while I focused on boot camps and nutritional consultations. On Sundays, we had outdoor boot camp sessions at the Jains' lawn that had a jogging track, followed by weekly nutrition strategy discussions over breakfast. It was my favourite time, and I began to relax.

By January 2010, after a year of training with Virtus, the Jains saw significant transformations.

'You finally look like the fit director of a fitness firm,' I teased myself.

12

WALKING THE TIGHTROPE OF LIFE

Baby Virtus had grown into a toddler when I found myself back in the maintenance phase of treatment. Despite the business running smoothly, the oral chemotherapy drugs led to drug-induced jaundice, and I was admitted to Lilavati once again. The ten days in the hospital were a stark reminder that I was still fighting cancer and walking a tightrope between life and death.

After almost a month, I recovered and returned to work, but Dr Bhave's words about finding a bone marrow donor lingered on my mind. I had neglected this critical aspect in my excitement about the business. I tried to find a match in the family, but Ammi was not a match, and Firoz was only a half-match.

Dr Bhave referred Firoz to Dr Shashikant Apte at Sahyadri Hospital, Pune, but the latter refused to proceed with a haploidentical bone marrow transplant, citing the low success rates. The other option was to find a complete match from an unrelated donor, known as a Match Unrelated Donor (M.U.D.) transplant.

Lying in the hospital bed, writhing in pain, I wondered if I would survive until the doctors found a suitable technology for transplants. 'Would there ever be a day when I could talk about this cancer without worrying about it?' I asked my spirit. Would I live to say, 'I had this cancer back then, much like I had a cold that winter?'

* * *

As a fitness enthusiast, I idolised Bruce Lee and Jackie Chan and would eagerly spend my precious Rs 2.50 to watch their movies in cinema halls. In Class VII, I stumbled upon an advertisement for Kung Fu classes in my neighbourhood and knew I had to join. When I told Felix sir, the coach, that I wanted to learn how to fight, he put me to the test. In just 90 seconds, I was beaten black and blue, but surprisingly, I enjoyed it. I knew I had to hide my bruises from Ammi, so I wore a full-sleeved T-shirt and namaz pyjamas.

I watched senior students practise animal techniques and asked Felix sir when I would learn them. He challenged me to do 1,500 push-ups before asking again! Undeterred, I eagerly worked towards the goal, and within a year, I managed 1,502 push-ups! Felix sir raised the bar, and I followed a rigorous schedule to participate in sub-junior-level competitions. With practice and determination, I climbed the ranks and found myself in state-level full-contact combats by Class IX.

Years later, as I lay in a hospital bed fighting cancer, I realised the true meaning of my first Kung Fu lesson. Martial arts are not just about combat, but an art form that requires patient endurance. Cancer may have beaten me up, but I refused to give up. I had no choice but to keep pushing and trying new techniques to stay alive.

I Can Do It

As a child, running was always my escape. It allowed me to indulge in 'me-time' and find freedom outside of my tiny home. But it wasn't until later in life, after being isolated in a hospital for hours, that I realised why I had always been drawn to long-distance endurance training. Running and cycling became my meditation and a way to prepare myself for the challenges life would throw my way.

I thought back to my daily routine as a child. Waking up at 4.30 a.m., running out to wake up my friends, doing drills or playing football at Chandivali playground, and then running back to make it home by 6.30 a.m. I had just enough time to shower, brush my teeth, have breakfast and start running again to get to school by 7 a.m. My school was only 1.2 kilometres away, and I could run there in just five minutes. The discipline I learned from this routine was what was helping me fight my current battle with cancer.

Although I wasn't a great student, I loved going to school because it had a 100-metre playground where I could run around. My Ammi would lock the door after lunch to ensure I studied, but I would sneak away to do push-ups and crunches. At 4 p.m., I could finally run again, playing gully cricket or school football. I was good enough to be noticed at the school level, and I was even the volleyball captain, leading my team to victory in every match.

Now, as a successful fitness consultant and business owner, I think back to my PT teacher, Anita ma'am, and sports sir,

Mr Warke, who would be proud of my accomplishments. But the voice within me always reminded me that there is still more to achieve, urging me to run the Comrades Marathon.

After my seventh round of chemotherapy, Dr Bhave gave me the good news that I was in remission once again! But I still had to wait five years to ensure the cancer didn't come back. In the meantime, I continued to work on my fitness and my business, Virtus Wellness. Long-distance cycling became my new passion, with the aim to cover a minimum distance of 60 kilometres and a maximum of 100 kilometres.

Life steadily improved, and I grew stronger and fitter. Although I still used to fall sick often due to my developing immune system, I was determined to keep pushing forward. I knew that discipline and perseverance were the keys to success, and I was ready for whatever challenges lay ahead.

13

LIFE'S PERFECT, UNTIL YET ANOTHER RELAPSE

During a cycling journey in 2013, I noticed mild swelling in my testicular region but ignored it as it didn't hurt much. I was preoccupied with thoughts of a short trip to Abu Dhabi to attend the upcoming Abu Dhabi International Triathlon. I loved the idea of swimming, cycling and running continuously for either the 113-kilometre or the 226-kilometre race.

I booked my tickets and planned to stay with my brother Firoz for a week, meet athletes, and learn more about triathlons. However, the pain and swelling in my testicles increased, but I ignored it and continued my fitness routine. Eventually, I felt an abnormal hardness around the area, and the fear of a possible tumour crept in.

Within two years of my first visit to Dr Bhave, I returned as the pain and swelling worsened. After a thorough examination, he referred me to a urologist in Lilavati. The urologist diagnosed me with testicular cancer and advised a biopsy to determine the type of cancer! I was devastated to hear this news after being declared cancer-free previously. I had to undergo chemotherapy again and again, driving me insane to the point where I wanted to scream! When will this stop, I asked the Gods!

* * *

With my tickets to Abu Dhabi booked, I asked Dr Bhave, 'Is it urgent, or can I start treatment in seven days?'

He replied with a reassuring smile, 'Go ahead and enjoy.'

Firoz was the first to know about my testicular relapse, which dampened our vacation mood. But once I settled in Abu Dhabi, we had a blast for the entire week. The preparation, distance and international rigour of the Triathlon left me impressed, and I wistfully told Firoz, 'How I would love to participate sometime.' Firoz smiled and said, 'God willing, you will, but first deal with this new roadblock.'

Once back in Mumbai, I immediately went for a biopsy, which confirmed acute lymphoblastic leukaemia (A.L.L.) relapse in my testicles. The chemotherapy protocols began for the third time, and this time they were more aggressive. Dr Bhave suggested inserting a chemotherapy port under my skin near the chest, which could administer the drugs without repeated pricking. The challenge was to keep it clean to avoid any infection.

As the sessions progressed, Dr Bhave emphasised the importance of finding a bone marrow match. I had forgotten about it, yet again. 'It's mandatory now,' Dr Bhave said, stressing each word slowly and clearly. 'You need a bone marrow transplant.'

Time To Meet the Marrow

Four months later, I achieved remission again. Though still on medication, I had zero malignant cell count. In August 2013, I took the initiative to meet Dr Shashikant Apte in Pune, bringing along Nitin Rane and my entire medical file dating back to 2004.

Firoz had previously visited Dr Apte in 2009, but the response was negative. However, with advancements in medical science, Dr Apte was confident this time. 'Start finding a donor. If we can find a full match, it's great. If not, we can go for a haploidentical transplant,' he said. He had successfully worked on several cases of haploidentical transplants, and I was determined to add my name to the list of success stories.

'The transplant is costly,' Dr Bhave said softly. 'Obtaining cells from an Indian donor will cost approximately Rs 8 lakh ($9700), while an American donor will cost about Rs 48–50 lakh (about $60,000). A European donor will cost around Rs 18–20 lakh ($25,000). Furthermore, the transplant operation takes approximately a month and costs roughly Rs 25 lakh ($30,000). After the transplant, there will be a two-year upkeep duration, and you should set aside around Rs 15 lakh (about $18,000) to combat any severe infection during this period.'

I quickly calculated the costs and realized I was staring at the total of about Rs 1 crore ($120,000).

'I will start searching for a donor,' I responded with conviction. I had come so far that I couldn't quit now. 'I will arrange for the funds,' I told myself.

In the previous few years, I had accomplished my business objectives. I purchased a flat in Andheri East, Mumbai. I was confident that I could collect roughly Rs 80–90 lakh ($1,10,000) by selling it, enough to begin the transplant and manage any major difficulties that might arise. My doctors and I started looking for a bone marrow donor.

However, the Indian bone marrow donor registry had a meagre list with no matches. We scoured the European registry, but again, no match. Three months had already passed, and it was November. We turned to the US registry, but it was already the Thanksgiving season, and donors were unlikely to show up. I needed the transplant quickly. Dr Apte decided to proceed with the haploidentical transplant with Firoz being the bone marrow donor. He called me in for a check-up only to discover that I was physically weak and not ready for the transplant. 'You have a two-month window. We will do it in January. Surviving the bone marrow transplant procedure will be easier on your body if you are fit,' he stated bluntly. It was the best news I had heard in a long time.

* * *

Getting fit was my top priority before the bone marrow transplant. I promised to enter the transplant room as fit as possible, which required investment in my betterment. Cycling was my chosen exercise, but a carbon bike was too expensive. A pre-owned triathlon bike at Rs 75,000 plus (about $900) suited my budget. I set off the next day from Andheri to Bandra and back. What used to feel like a fun game now seemed like a slow struggle. I shopped online for indoor training equipment and rode twice a week outdoors and once a week indoors. Short bursts at the gym filled the rest of my days.

By December, I completed all required blood tests and paid the deposit for the bone marrow transplant at Sahyadri Hospital in Pune, scheduled for 7 January 2014. The procedure was to last six months with recovery time in Pune. With just a month left, I needed to rent an apartment near the hospital and adjust to a new city.

Life Transplants to Pune

On a Friday evening, I embarked on a journey to Pune. Nainesh Shah, a Terraform Realty client of Virtus, had referred me to an estate agent who had arranged a couple of apartment viewings. As my car twisted and turned up the winding roads that overlooked deep valleys, the sun began to set over the Western Ghats.

The feeling of déjà vu set in, as I had started a similar house hunt near Lilavati Hospital back in 2004. Now, ten years later, I found myself searching for an apartment near another hospital in a different city. Life had come full circle, and the cancer that I thought I would recover from in a few years continued to gnaw at me, devouring me from the inside. This time, the beast's teeth were the sharpest they had ever been.

As I approached Pune, I couldn't help but wonder if it would be life's final destination for me.

* * *

Finding the perfect apartment was no easy feat. It had to be clean, hygienic, and far from any construction sites. Plus, it had to be close enough to Sahyadri in case of emergencies. After much searching, I found a flat that seemed promising and met with the owners, a lawyer and a doctor couple.

But there was one problem—I was bald with no eyebrows or lashes and wearing a mask. The owner asked me why I needed the flat and I explained my situation, battling leukaemia and in need of a place near the hospital for a bone marrow transplant.

His immediate response shocked me: 'Sorry, not this flat.' The estate agent later explained that they may have thought my illness would bring misfortune or bad luck. I was prevented from renting other apartments on religious grounds. After a month of searching and viewing eighteen properties, I never expected it to be so difficult to find a place in a satellite city like Pune. With barely any time left, I headed back to Mumbai, the long shadows of the night casting over the mountains.

Angels Keep a Watch

My angels came to my rescue once again. On a Monday morning, Dharmesh Jain transferred some funds into my account. 'Let me know when you need more. Return it when you can. Don't worry about it if you can't,' he said. I was overwhelmed with gratitude.

More good news followed. During the last weekend of 2013, I met the nineteenth landlord in Pune whose only concern was the rent. Finally, I found someone who didn't care about my disease or religion as the landlord lived in the USA, and his friend had the power of attorney.

After so many trials and tribulations, I had finally found

an understanding and accommodating landlord. We signed the deal, and the three-bedroom apartment was mine for the duration of my stay in Pune.

My estate agent went above and beyond his duties, managing all the paperwork, arranging fumigation, cooking gas and even helping install small fittings. The apartment was already semi-furnished, and he found people to clean and sanitise everything.

With the finances and location sorted, all that was left was for me to up my fitness game.

Pune was a done deal, sealed and signed.

We headed back to Mumbai to pack. There, I utilised the remaining winter mornings to cycle and run and by 31 December 2013, I had cycled non-stop for 102 kilometres. Finally, I was fit again, but it was disheartening to know that I would lose it all when I returned to the hospital within a week. However, I had no time to mope. I had to pack up my life again, this time leaving Mumbai for a long period. It was the first time I was leaving my hometown, and surprisingly, I felt a twinge of sadness. I never realized how much I loved the city.

'It's only six months and I'll be back,' I promised myself. I tried to feel excited about staying in a new city, but it only lasted for two hours.

Off to Pune for Six Months

On 5 January, we said goodbye to Mumbai and drove towards Pune. The city was bustling as usual, but the car was silent. As we reached our new home in Kothrud, a Pune suburb, the sun was about to set. The interiors were clean, quiet and residential. Pune's air was already cleaner and crisper, and the streets were well-maintained.

Our estate agent had done an excellent job, and the apartment was ready for us to move in. Firoz began unpacking while Ammi and I went for a walk to find grocery shops, chemists and restaurants. This time, it was Ammi who was the stronger one.

'Experience, even negative ones, can build you,' I reminded myself. Ammi and Firoz ordered in for the night, and I cooked myself some eggs for dinner. We all agreed to call it a night as the air was getting chilly. We dozed off, much happier than we were in the morning. The excitement I was looking for that morning had finally arrived.

The next morning in our new kitchen, I took charge of breakfast while Firoz and Ammi began organising the apartment. We spent the morning in a happy buzz, sorting out power points, geysers, air-conditioning, and most importantly, finding daily help.

Fortunately, we found our angels in Pune. One of my Virtus employees had a cousin sister named Manju in the city, and her best friend Nazia came to our aid. Nazia sent over lunches and dinners for the entire week and promised to do so until we were settled in. She also helped us find a helper, which eased the load off Ammi and made settling down in Pune much easier.

* * *

At that moment, my life felt like a stick fight from my childhood. The Lakshmi Narayan temple, located in the backyard of my chawl, stood green and serene. The ground surrounding the temple had tall coconut and Ashoka trees and was the site of a political *shakha* (bureau) where young boys were trained in stick fighting. I would sit on the high boundary walls, legs dangling and listening to the instructors speak Sanskrit slogans.

One day, I mustered the courage to approach the instructor and request stick-fighting lessons. He agreed, and after my training was over, he even paid a social visit to my home. He was surprised to see no temples or portraits depicting any gods, and Ammi explained that we were Muslims. The instructor found it amusing since the training he provided was meant for Hindu boys in political alignment with the bureau. However, he was pleased with my progress and even referred to me as 'Shivraj' because he could never get my name right.

After a decade, I had regained my fitness and was once again at my best. But just like in a stick fight, the following day I would go in for a procedure that would leave me fragile once again. The stick would turn the other way, even before I could blink.

14

THE D-DAY

7 January 2014. On that clear winter morning, I chose to stand alone on the balcony instead of joining my family. With a crucial transplant coming up, I didn't want to waste any time. I took in the fresh air and direct sunlight, and watched the day begin in Pune with birds chirping and a cold breeze flitting through the dappled morning sunlight. It felt like standing on the peak of a mountain, with the past on one side and the future on the other, but I had no foothold.

It was time to say goodbye to Ammi at 8 a.m. '*Achha ho ke wapas aana* (come back healed),' she blessed me with a smile. Despite feeling wrung up inside, she was holding herself well. I was proud of her, but my own emotions were difficult to manage. The transplant was a critical and life-threatening process, and I didn't know if I would see her again.

Firoz and I took a rickshaw to the hospital as neither of us wanted to drive. This time, I had Firoz to chat with and share my thoughts and feelings. He would stay with us for just ten more days before returning to Oman. During the twenty-minute journey, we discussed important yet trivial matters, like arranging for house help and skirting around the ifs and if-nots.

Finally, we arrived at Sahyadri, where we were to be admitted. The doctors had warned us that a 24-hour attendant was mandatory and that the transplant procedure would make me extremely weak. They also informed us that the donor must be present much before the attendant.

* * *

Dr Aditi Joshi, Dr Apte's assistant, greeted us with a smile as we arrived at the hospital lobby. She efficiently guided us through the admission process and led us to the haematology department, which was located near Deccan Gymkhana, a well-known club in Pune.

'Today, we will insert a mandatory catheter,' Dr Aditi explained with a smile. 'It's like a central line, to make the patient's life a little easier.'

After changing into the blue-checked hospital uniform, we were instructed not to eat or drink anything until the catheter insertion surgery at 6 p.m. We passed the time enjoying the view until I was taken to the icy-cold waiting room near the operation theatre. I felt a chill and requested a blanket, which was quickly provided.

The surgeon arrived and administered general anaesthesia. They started with the lumbar puncture procedure to test for cancer cells in the cerebrospinal fluid. Once this was done, the chemotherapy drug was injected followed by the insertion of the Hickman's catheter through the jugular vein in my neck. The procedure took around 45 minutes, and I dozed off.

When I woke up four hours later, I was fully conscious and allowed to start drinking fluids. By 10 p.m., I was transferred to the bone marrow transplant room where I could see Firoz waiting patiently through the glass windows.

We ate a fresh homemade meal in silence, using the hospital steriliser to sanitise the spoons and plates. I asked Firoz to go home as there was no point in my mother being alone in a new city at night. He agreed, promising to come back with breakfast the next morning.

* * *

8 January 2014. I was in one of the two pressure-controlled transplant rooms with the reception desk facing us. Firoz had already arrived and gone through the necessary sterilisation process, including changing clothes and footwear, and wearing a mask. He brought breakfast with him, but before entering the room, he steamed his cutlery at the first station for 20 minutes.

My favourite meal of eggs, rotis and a cup of tea arrived, but they had to go through the steriliser too, which made them overcooked and less appetising. But following the protocol was crucial for my safety.

It was surreal to think that my life depended on eating mushy eggs and rotis.

Dr Apte entered the room with his entourage, wearing a broad smile and cheerfully greeting me, 'Good morning!' He introduced Dr Girish and Sister Aditi, who, along with two to three specially trained nurses per shift, would be taking care of me during my stay in the transplant room. He assured me that I could take up to a month here in my temporary home, which had HEPA air-conditioning filters to prevent fungus and pollutants. The pressure-controlled room ensured that outside air would not enter, and anyone with even a hint of a cold or cough would be barred from entering.

When Dr Apte announced, 'Within one hour, we will start conditioning,' little did I know that conditioning was a painful process. Toxic chemotherapy drugs were injected into me to eradicate my bone marrow, a process that took six days. Firoz also had his conditioning, which was comparatively easier. He received Filgrastim injections twice a day to increase his white blood cell count. We both followed a strict diet and were not allowed to eat outside food to avoid the risk of infection, which could prove fatal for me since my bone marrow was completely eradicated during conditioning.

After my body wash that night, I was not allowed to move much until the catheter was in place. In the opposite transplant room, a child was recovering from a full-match bone marrow transplant, and I watched the mother nurse her child while following Dr Apte's precautions. Meanwhile, my home front was taken care of by Nazia, who arranged my meals, and Ammi, who was comfortable in her new environment. Maya, a colleague at Virtus, had relatives in Pune and came to visit, while Manju was scheduled to come for a week. Nitin Rane, my manager, proved to be a supportive brother, and ran the business smoothly.

My life right now seemed to echo the camaraderie at the Comrades marathon. Friends, family and even strangers motivated and volunteered to help, fostering trust and positivity. I could focus on my battle in the transplant room without any worries about my home and business fronts. Firoz had even put on some weight, and I was sure the duties of travelling and marrow donations would get him back in shape.

* * *

16 January 2014. Zero Day, the day of the bone marrow transplant, marked my rebirth. I was getting a haploidentical peripheral blood stem cell transplant, and like every transplant patient, I felt like a newborn baby kept in an incubator before the transplant began.

Firoz had already been admitted overnight, and the donation process had been completed. With filgrastim injections, his WBC count had reached above 35,000. The average for a healthy individual is just 4,000. All the other cells had been returned to him, and he was now resting.

It was my turn now. I started receiving the marrow, and it felt no different from a blood transfusion. The process was comfortable and took no more than 90 minutes. As I closed my eyes, I visualised myself healed. However, I knew that the story wasn't over yet; it had just begun.

* * *

From Day Zero, I was put on high doses of mandatory immunity-suppressant drugs. Dr Apte warned me, 'The first six months will be extremely crucial. If the transplant fails, it'll happen mostly within the first six months. Also, you risk fatal complications. Graft Versus Host Disease (GVHD) is much needed for a successful transplant, but you'll have to fight it too."

I was aware of the drill and had to be conscious of hygiene, food, water and even the air I breathed. Moreover, I was on high doses of antibiotics through intravenous tubes and immunoglobin injections for the next six months.

Firoz, the donor, was instructed that he could resume his routine within two days to a week at the maximum. 'Donor safety is the top priority,' Dr Apte emphasised as he signed Firoz's discharge form.

Firoz experienced side effects of filgrastim injections; he had been nauseous for a whole week. He felt better two days after the transplant was over and by the seventh day, he was completely fine. He headed back to Oman to work the next day as he had extended his leave by fifteen days and couldn't push it anymore.

Firoz Taught Me Biking, Cycling and Gave Me My Life

Firoz, seven years my senior, taught me cycling in just one day. We and our friends rented cycles from a shop for 30 minutes to an hour, exploring the city like it was our playground. The 50 paise rate was perfect, but it increased to a steep 1.50 rupees soon after. We had to start saving up.

Then, our neighbour Vikas got a new cycle. Thanks to Firoz, I was chosen to teach Viki how to ride. I had the awesome, sporty, and fast BSA SLR bike as my ride and coach.

Years later, Firoz bought a Hero Honda motorbike when he got his first job at a petrochemical company. He used it, and when the time came, Firoz taught me how to ride it. The bike was very special to me.

Now, it was Firoz again who gave me my life. I lay back, grateful for his presence in my life.

* * *

In my super-hygienic, filtered transplant room, I lay waiting alongside the doctors. Days two through six were a blur of pathology tests, injections and a long list of medications that filled my plate. I was monitored closely for signs of GVHD, a potentially life-threatening complication that often arises after haploidentical bone marrow transplants. With my white cell count hovering at 100 instead of the average of 4,000, the risk of infection was high.

Sleep eluded me and I resorted to sleeping pills. Within two weeks, I had lost a staggering 17 kilos and was too weak to walk to the washroom without difficulty. As I drifted in and out of consciousness, memories flooded my mind. By Day 15, bone pain had overtaken my body, and my normally sprightly spirit had abandoned me. But I knew I had to keep climbing.

The word took me back to the hills of Pereirawadi where Firoz and I would race up the hill with our friends, huffing and puffing and our bodies screaming in pain. At the summit, we would savour wild berries and have picnics with bhajiyas and vada pavs. Evenings came too soon, and we would run back 'as fast as possible' through the forest area before dark.

But now, despite the super-bright, super-clean room, I felt the darkness creeping in. Dr Apte's worry lines only added to the gloom. I yearned for the polluted 'fresh' air, the wind, and the silence of Pereirawadi. Where was the peace I had felt on that rock? Had it gone up in smoke with my spirit, abandoned? Thoughts raced through my mind.

On day nineteen, post-transplant, my white cell count finally rose from a measly 100 to a hopeful 600. The next day, it was 900, and within just one more day, it hit 1,100. Dr Apte and his assistants breathed a sigh of relief. 'In three to four days, we can move you to the private ward to get you acclimated to normal air,' Dr Apte informed me. Who knew we needed to adapt to the air we breathe? I thought back to high-altitude acclimatisation. The private ward was fumigated, and I would be there for at least another four days.

Breathing Freely Again

First February 2014 was an iconic day. The newborn was being shifted out of the incubator into regular air, and I had to learn to breathe normally again too. As I left the bone marrow transplant room for the private ward, the change felt drastic. Suddenly, there was a lot of noise. Doctors, nurses and staff entered the room, speaking to me. Although my family had visited me through the window while I was in isolation, it had been nothing more than a few waves. After 21 days of silence and seclusion, I was delighted to hear the sounds of traffic from outside!

Another four days in the ward and I seemed to be doing well in normal air.

15

FINALLY, THE DISCHARGE

5 February 2014. My discharge form was signed and, boy, was I ecstatic! Finally, I would be going home and reuniting with Ammi. I felt like a kid returning home from boarding school.

The hospital lobby was crowded with people. This normal crowd would have irritated almost anyone, but it was exciting to me. I realised how lonely I had been up there. As I stepped out of the hospital, the sun's rays hit my skin. I felt Pune's warmth, took deep breaths of its polluted but fresh air through my mask, and savoured the moment. The sunlight looked different, and a sense of newness pervaded my being.

I had conquered. I was confident that I had beaten cancer. The battle was over. However, as I stepped into the driver's seat, I knew the war had just begun. The first 100 days post-transplant were the most crucial. Bone marrow rejection could happen within six months, and any organ rejection or even any serious infection could quickly wipe me out.

Still, I decided to enjoy the moment. I felt light-hearted, almost tizzy, enjoying each press of the accelerator, each change of the gear in my hand. Life felt like a new journey from the hospital to my new house. Having Nitin beside me doubled my joy. 'I wouldn't be here if Firoz weren't,' I said, finally expressing the gratitude that had been building up inside me for over a month.

It had been a roller-coaster month for both brothers. Pune's constant honking, auto-rickshaws stopping mid-way, and reckless bikers did not irritate me in the least. I had the wheel in my hands and was heading home. Nothing could disturb this happy feeling. I had won.

* * *

'I'm unrecognisable,' I said as I walked into my home. My mother's eyes widened as she took in my appearance or lack thereof. Tears welled up in both our eyes as we hugged each other tightly. It had been a difficult time for me, but my mother had been my rock.

'What will you eat?' she asked, a smile breaking through the tears. 'Your favourite biryani is already waiting for you.' We laughed, relieved to have something normal to look forward to.

Ten years of chemotherapy seemed like a distant memory now, pushed aside by the intensity of the past month's transplant treatment. I was grateful to be back home, no longer confined to a hospital bed.

I remembered a quote by boxing legend Muhammad Ali: 'I only start counting when it starts hurting.' This experience had certainly been painful, but I had made it through to the other side.

* * *

Sipping my morning tea on the balcony, my gaze landed on a blue kite, faded with time, fluttering amidst the trees. Memories of my childhood filled my mind, of chasing kites and climbing trees to retrieve them, emerging unrecognisable and only requiring a simple bath to clean up. But now, I could only wait and watch, unable to participate due to my physical limitations.

I thought back to my classmate Sylvia, a math genius who I struggled to learn from, while her brother Godfrey taught me the art of kite-flying effortlessly. Life offered me both lessons, but I accepted only one, rejecting the other. Perhaps destiny was trying to teach me to stretch my physical limits and endure pain.

Cut and bruised, I had to pull myself together once again. Just like in kite-flying, I had to master the technique of letting go before pulling taut. Even pain was a reminder of the good that can come from it.

As kids, we couldn't afford new kites, so we chased the ones whose threads were cut and who made trees their temporary residences. The dusty trees and mingled sweat and dirt left us unrecognisable. Now, again, I had changed so much—all bones, no hair, no lashes, weighing no more than 57.5 kilos.

But just like in kite-flying, the chase was often long and hard. And just like then, I had to learn to master my physical self and endure pain.

* * *

Despite it being almost the end of February, Pune's winter felt too severe for a transplant patient like me. Bundled up in bed with blankets, sweaters and socks, I reminisced about my childhood in Mumbai, where winters meant Christmas vacations and early morning adventures with friends. We would collect wood, cardboard and paper, and light campfires to keep warm at the Chandivali playground.

But now, in Pune, I was too weak to even handle my daily routine without help. I had been entrusted with an important book to record my treatments, medicines and meals each day. Manju's cousin sister, Meenu, had come to help for the next seven days. I even hired Vijay, a housekeeping attendant at Virtus, to stay with me in Pune at least until May, as I needed someone to constantly be around to support me with walking, do household errands and accompany me while driving. I could drive but could not walk without support.

Every Tuesday and Friday, I made my way to Sahyadri Hospital. Going to Lilavati had been a delightful escape from being cooped up at home, but this time it was a different story. My body was simply too weak, leaving me gasping for air most of the time. The routine pathology tests at Sahyadri were a gruelling experience that required me to wait for two hours for the results. Most days, I couldn't even sit up and would resort to lying down in the casualty department.

Hospital food and water were off-limits for me, so I carried boiled water and a box of sterilised food that contained a few biscuits and snacks. I felt like a newborn baby all over again!

'The haemoglobin count is still low, that's why you're having trouble breathing,' explained Dr Aditi, offering some quick reassurance, 'But it will improve soon.'

Luckily, the rest of the reports came back normal, and I was allowed to go home. It was like a baby's day out! Thankfully, February passed without any major incidents.

* * *

March was not kind to me as I battled with two setbacks—fungal pneumonia and a CMV infection—which were common complications for patients with a weakened immune system like me. The pneumonia was a close call and I had to be readmitted for treatment. As soon as I was discharged, I was hit with a CMV infection. This one was particularly dangerous for transplant patients, so I had to receive strong antibiotics through injections at Sahyadri twice daily. The stubborn infection took 21 long days to clear, but thankfully, I emerged victorious. However, the one thing that could confirm the success of my transplant, GVHD, was still nowhere in sight.

100 Days Done

3 May 2014. Despite the fevers, infections and weakness, three months had passed, and I was grateful to be alive and home most of the time. I had overcome the most crucial stage post-transplant, the 100-day milestone. 'Time to get life back on track,' I said to Ammi.

On Day 101, I called Dr Apte to ask permission to start indoor exercises. He allowed me light exercises but strictly prohibited me from going outdoors. It wasn't easy. Even a few crunches, 30 seconds of jumps, and a few spot jogs sent my heart racing, and I felt dizzy with my pressure dropping. But I didn't let this physical weakness demotivate me. I am determined to run the Comrades Marathon in 2015, a dream that has been incubated for over a decade, and now there are no more reasons to wait. The countdown to becoming the fittest ever has begun.

Day 103

I am going strong. My heart is pumping and my limbs are aching, but I'm loving it. This is what I've been longing for—getting fit again. Dr Apte gave me a glimmer of hope, saying I could start walking outdoors after 120 days, but only if I felt up to it. I made up my mind to stick to that schedule.

Every day, I added one more minute to my indoor workout routine and gradually increased it by three minutes each week. The progress was slow but steady, and it helped improve my overall endurance levels.

Day 120

I had reached a new milestone in my fitness journey—working out non-stop for 15 minutes without gasping. It felt like a marathon feat. Dr Apte had permitted me to visit a nearby park, but the road was undulating, and I was not confident dealing with the traffic. Despite feeling weak and tired, I decided to take small, cautious steps and entered the park gate. Resting for a few minutes, I began to walk, but I had to stop every 100 metres due to exhaustion and tightness in my calves.

Watching four other men take continuous rounds of the park, I told myself, 'Before leaving Pune, I will walk continuously for five kilometres.' With only a month left in Pune, I continued my training—indoor workouts in the morning and outdoors in the evening, slowly increasing my endurance levels. My haemoglobin count improved, and so did my ability to sustain cardiovascular exercise.

Back to the Future

My past gave me the courage to face the future. I used to run five kilometres to play near Sahar International Airport and back. Security around the airport wasn't as strict then. We created a special airport game by pushing the luggage trolley up the ramp to the main entrance. All our friends, except one, would climb onto the trolley, and the one friend who was on the ground would push the trolley down the slope! Each took turns to push the trolley. The one who pushed the hardest and made the trolley go the fastest was the winner.

Back then, it was nothing more than childhood love for speed. It was unbridled, and nobody thought local kids having fun were a nuisance or a threat. The security guards at the gate would often give us water and some health tips for free. Arun Pandey, one of the guards, a fitness enthusiast and a regular at the local gym, advised me, 'Soak a handful of green or brown channa (chickpeas) at night. As soon as you wake up, drink that water first. Then, munch the channa raw before you come out early in the morning. It will increase your stamina and endurance.'

I followed his advice religiously for many months. After all, I was impressed by Mr Pandey's athletic physique, crisply ironed clothes, and army-like, chest-out-tummy-in posture.

Blocked Jugular

I always thought my life was a marathon, but now it felt like a hurdle race with obstacles at every turn. However, I kept making progress every day, and my fitness levels started to improve. I was starting to feel in control once again.

In April, during my regular tests at Sahyadri Hospital, the nurse couldn't get a blood sample from my catheter, which was blocked because of a clot. Dr Apte decided to remove it the next day.

On 2 April, I was back in the day-care unit, faced with two choices: to try to remove the catheter under local anaesthesia or to use general anaesthesia, which would require an overnight stay. I chose the former and prepared myself for the pain. I did not want to spend one more night in a hospital.

The procedure was excruciatingly painful, as the catheter had become a part of my body due to tissue growth around it. Dr Apte finally managed to remove it after about 40 minutes of trying, leaving me soaked in perspiration.

Once the bleeding wound was cleaned, I was allowed to leave with the instruction not to bathe for the next 48 hours. I was finally catheter-free!

Not Taking the Easy Way

'I'll reach my goal, Ammi. I won't take the easy way out,' I declared. The lesson of not taking shortcuts had been ingrained in me since childhood. Growing up in a chawl, I had friendly neighbours and friends but also encountered the darker side of gangs and gangsters. We heard stories of police brutality and shopkeepers paying 'protection money' to these people. Bollywood movies, particularly gangster films like Arjun and Ankush, were popular and influential.

One day, a boy named Pramod showed off his expensive watches and chocolates, claiming that he didn't need money to buy them, one only needed to be smart. He had learned successful tricks from his elder brother and challenged us to come along and learn. We all watched, fascinated, as Pramod entered a crowded grocery store and just walked out with a big bar of chocolate!

'You try it now,' he urged. Sridhar and I tried and failed

miserably with the shopkeeper spotting us and yelling. At that moment, both of us knew that we should have listened to our fear, even though we could not articulate it to be the voice of conscience back then.

We froze. Our parents were informed about our misdemeanour, and we were thoroughly thrashed at home! I learnt the hard way that discipline meant working for what you wanted. The incident taught me that taking the easy way out was never the right path.

As I grew older and learned about athletes using performance-enhancing drugs, I knew it was another form of taking the easy way out. Building a castle on weak foundations was bound to make the structure crumble eventually. Today, as I tried to run, I was grateful for that childhood lesson. Ambition is great, but it requires hard work to turn dreams into reality.

* * *

Determined to overcome cancer and regain my fitness, I set a goal to walk non-stop for five kilometres before leaving Pune for Mumbai. I pushed myself harder each day, just like my mother had done when she learned how to cook the labour-intensive biryani by travelling daily from our home in Saki Naka to a lunch-house in Vikhroli. Despite being a talented mehndi artist, she too continued to hone her skills by taking the train to her friend's place in Vikhroli when I was in Class 7.

Unlike my mother, I had to try even harder to achieve my goal of walking five kilometres. At that time, I could only manage one-and-a-half kilometres, and I knew I had a long way to go with limited time to reach my target. So, I stayed strict and firm in my resolve to push a little harder each day.

Fitness and Recovery Were Top Priorities

I jokingly told Nitin, 'The trainer needs a trainer.'

I remembered my table tennis days, fumbling around without a coach. When we moved to Kalyan, I hired Raj Kshatriya, a professional weight-training coach, to help me develop muscle and get a toned physique. Raj was knowledgeable and mature in his approach, recognising my endurance and egging me on to greater heights. I was able to do 1,000 squats in the gym and achieved my personal best of 3,500 squats in one go!

Raj pushed me further and asked me to try spot jogging for fat loss. Starting with just five minutes, I eventually worked my way up to spot-jogging for a full five hours! That was back in 2000. Now, I was the director of Virtus Wellness, a fitness company, and had to find my guru within myself.

That realisation helped me push even harder. And on 22 May 2014, I finally accomplished my goal of walking five kilometres non-stop. Goal achieved!

16

BACK TO MUMBAI'S NOISE AND LOVING IT!

25 May 2014. It was time to bid farewell to Pune. With better reports and steady progress, I felt like I had won the war against cancer. Dr Apte permitted me to return to Mumbai despite concerns about my GVHD. I decided to take the wheel myself and drive back with the help of Firoz, Nitin and Nainesh Shah's driver. Nitin and the car proved valuable, and I felt my life was back in the fast lane as we left Pune.

After a long day, we reached home in Mumbai and began unloading the two cars. Nitin had arranged for helpers to clean the house, and Zeenat, our house help, cooked a simple meal. I quickly sterilised the food and dined. We unpacked only essentials, leaving the rest for the next day.

I informed my Virtus team that things were back to normal, but I needed to disinfect the equipment before hitting the gym. As I lay down to rest, tired but happy, I was grateful to be back home and on my way to recovery.

2 June 2014. It was my first day at the gym. I cycled five kilometres, did light strength training, and stretched to cool down. The workout was slow and low impact, but it encouraged me. I called Dr Apte the next day with an exuberant plan, 'September 16 is my birthday. I want to get back to my old fitness level by then, and do 100 km of indoor cycling.'

'What exactly do you want to do?' asked Dr Apte, to which I replied, 'Before entering the transplant room, I could do 102 km of cycling.'

'Okay,' was his one-word response. But he warned me to do all the tests on time, check my vital parameters, and not stress too much as it could harm my immune system. 'Be very cautious, Shiraz. You have just completed five months after the bone marrow transplant. The first two years after the transplant are crucial.'

* * *

The very next day, my body was quick to remind me of Dr Apte's warnings. After cycling just five kilometres, I was sore and out of commission for the next three days. But I was determined not to give up. On the fourth day, I hit the gym again and stuck to a low-impact workout. I understood what Dr Apte meant by 'do not stress'—my body needed time to recover from all it had been through.

Despite the setback, I was confident in my birthday goal. 'My goals have the power to transform me,' I told Firoz as we sat around the dinner table that night.

GVHD Strikes

I had only been back in Mumbai for a week when I noticed some skin discolouration and black patches while bathing on a Sunday. Dr Apte requested some photos and quickly called back after seeing them. 'Come to Pune immediately,' he said, 'you finally have Graft Versus Host Disease.' The team had been waiting for this development for five months, which happened within a week of my return to Mumbai. I was annoyed that I had to take another break but relieved that the transplant was working. Emotionally confused, I went to Pune the next day.

Thankfully, I only had to stay one night at Sahyadri Hospital, where Dr Apte informed me that I would need steroids and regular medication for the next three to six months. He advised me to meet him once a month in Pune for pathology tests, while Dr Bhave would do regular physical examinations to check the progress of this disease, in common parlance known as GVHD. I returned to Mumbai the next day.

* * *

I had set my sights on cycling 100 kilometres, but the GVHD made it even more challenging. The side effects weakened me, made me prone to cramps, and left my skin sensitive and burning. Even my mouth was affected, making it difficult to eat or drink anything hot or cold. And the steroids only increased my cravings for sugary and salty foods, making it crucial to control my diet to avoid putting on weight and starting insulin. To manage my blood sugar better, I added more low-impact cardiovascular exercises to my routine.

But memories of the chawl and its festive foods, especially Ammi's biryani, made me nostalgic. I missed the Diwali sweets we would get from our neighbours. Rajesh, Sheetal and Shekhar's moms used to make lots of farsan snacks as well. Then there were the Catholic neighbours, Clifford's family and his mum, to whom all the chawl toddlers went to learn their alphabet. Christmas was all about marshmallows and the delicacy of kal kal. I used to gorge on rum cake, and Clifford would always indulge in Ammi's biryani during Eid.

* * *

Running didn't stop me then, and it couldn't stop me now. Dr Bhave checked on my progress once every 10 days and everything seemed to be going well.

After two more weeks of training, I decided to push a little harder, sticking to low-impact exercises. By the end of the third week, I could cycle for 25 kilometres without stopping.

Over the next four weeks, I gradually included a third cycling session each week, as well as regular walks in the nearby park, strength training to strengthen my lumbar region, and core workouts to help maintain my position while cycling.

Although my mind was strong, my body was still weak. My immunity was low and even a cold, cough, or sinusitis would derail my routine. However, I refused to stop my cycling routine, even if it meant skipping walks or strength training sometimes. The three cycling sessions each week were non-negotiable.

The steroids were taking a toll on my body. They made me weak, tired and sleep-deprived. By the end of July, I decided to do a test run. I had a month and a half left to achieve my goal of cycling 100 kilometres, so I attempted to cycle 50 kilometres non-stop by the end of the month.

I was confident that I could do it, having the stamina to ride about 25 kilometres per hour. Balancing my nutrition was critical, though, as I needed the right amount of hydration and carbohydrates to keep me going at the same pace for the entire journey.

On 31 July, I accomplished my goal of cycling 50 kilometres non-stop. I was weak and exhausted but thrilled to bits.

The next day, however, I came down with a viral fever.

Nearly There

Resting with nothing but my thumbs to twiddle, I set my sights on a new goal: cycling 65 kilometres non-stop. When I resumed cycling a week later, I struggled to reach the 50-kilometre mark, and by the time I hit 55 kilometres, my heart rate was skyrocketing, and I couldn't go any further.

If I was going to reach my goal of 65 kilometres by next week, I had to take urgent action. So, I made a new list:

- *Prioritise my nutrition.*
- *Practise breathing exercises every morning to improve my lung capacity.*
- *Dedicate 15–20 minutes of each day to meditation to sharpen my focus.*
- *Stay hydrated to keep my body balanced.*
- *Monitor my carbohydrate intake precisely and regularly.*

With these changes in place, I was determined to reach my goal of cycling 100 kilometres by my birthday on 16 September 16. And on 15 August, I hit my target of 65 kilometres of non-stop cycling, filled with excitement for what was to come.

On 16 August, I set a new goal of cycling 80 kilometres for the week.. Despite falling sick and missing four days of training, I managed to comfortably cycle 85 kilometres by the first week of September.

Pedalling to 100!

16 September 2014. It was a special birthday morning. Firoz had come down from Oman to celebrate with me. As I woke up at 6 a.m. and did my breathing exercises and meditation, I couldn't contain my excitement about cycling 100 kilometres that day.

It was going to be a long day—four hours of non-stop cycling. I packed a meal of boiled potatoes, steamed and sterilised, and several bottles of hydration. I loaded my car and sped off to the gym.

After a quick change, I briefed my senior staff, Roshan and Nilesh, about what I needed and at what time. I started riding at exactly 9 a.m. and aimed to maintain a pace of 25 km/hr. I kept track of my heart rate, hydration and carbohydrate intake every hour. At the 50-kilometre mark, I felt great. But my back started hurting at 60 km, and I had to slow down.

I hit the 65-kilometre mark, and my head and back were causing me acute pain acutely. I drank more water infused with electrolytes and kept going. By the time I reached 68 km, I regained my energy, and riding became comfortable. But at 87 km, my heart rate spiked, and I had to slow down again.

Then, at 1 p.m. sharp, I completed my goal of cycling 100 kilometres non-stop! Firoz and my entire team walked in to cheer me on. It was the ultimate victory!

Years later, that photograph stayed with me as a reminder to push myself further in every marathon. The Comrades were calling. But for now, it was time to cut the cake and eat it too!

PART III

Mind Over Matter

17

MIND ON COMRADES

I lay in bed, recovering from the gruelling 100-kilometre non-stop cycling adventure. It was well past midnight, yet sleep eluded me. My thoughts were fixated on the Comrades Marathon.

In my mind, I drew a connection between the Comrades and my personal history intertwined with India. The echoes of Prime Minister Jawaharlal Nehru's iconic speech at the Red Fort in New Delhi on 16 August 1947 reverberated within me. His words, 'winning back what is ours', resonated deeply. But for me, it was a different kind of victory I sought. I yearned to reclaim what was truly mine: my body, my spirit, my life.

Having lived my days from one chemotherapy cycle to the next, I longed for a new rhythm. I aspired to live from 'one marathon to the next'. Now that I had triumphed over the arduous 100-kilometre challenge, I felt primed for the Comrades and the demanding training it entailed. I was prepared to confront the pain head-on.

Perhaps sports was in my genes; my father was one of the best hockey players in his school and college back in Uttar Pradesh. When he moved to Mumbai, he let it all drift in the routines of daily survival.

I will make my father proud by running the Comrades. A sense of exuberance enveloped me.

The Brown Canvas Shoes

As I knotted the laces of my high-performance trainers, a wave of nostalgia washed over me, transporting me back to my modest beginnings in the world of running. The vivid recollection of Bata's trusty brown canvas shoes and their distinct aroma flooded my mind. Those shoes were my steadfast companions, enduring countless running sessions, football matches, and daring tree-climbing escapades.

Then, during my seventh-grade athletic pursuits, I upgraded to the more sophisticated and comfortable Bullet shoes, funded mostly by my hard-earned savings and timely assistance from Ammi. They came at nearly double the price but managed to endure an astonishing six months, a testament to their remarkable durability.

Now, as I geared up for the formidable challenge of the Comrades race, I drew inspiration from the unwavering resilience of those shoes. I resolved to embody their enduring spirit.

Make no mistake, the Comrades race is no walk in the park. Stretching across a gruelling 90 kilometres, it presents an array of uphill battles, aggressive ascents and mind-boggling descents. To meet the stringent qualifying criteria of completing a full marathon within four hours and fifty minutes, I needed unwavering strength. This demanded meticulous planning and a laser-like focus on nourishing my body with wholesome seasonal foods to fortify my immune system.

Importance of a Healthy Diet

As I was growing up, the importance of a nutritious diet was ingrained in me long before I became a trained nutritionist. Now, as I geared up for the exhilarating challenge of the Comrades race, I fully grasped the significance of meticulously planning my meals to ensure peak performance.

I owe a tremendous debt of gratitude to my mother for fostering a healthy routine in me from an early age. Tea and coffee were strictly off my menu. Before embarking on my 4 a.m. runs, I would indulge in a glass of milk, occasionally mixed with packaged malts or a drizzle of honey, accompanied by a few biscuits. It was the act of drinking itself that held my focus, rather than the taste of the contents in my cup.

Upon returning from my run, breakfast was non-negotiable before dashing off to school. I would savour my glass of milk alongside a couple of wheat chapatis and a two-egg omelette cooked in ghee. Butter, jam and bread were reserved for times of exceptional hunger and held little allure for me. The delightful crispness of brun pav remained a favourite of my mother and uncle. This nourishing breakfast, following an active morning, provided sustained energy throughout the school day.

In our household, there was always a matka, an earthen pot, for storing our daily drinking water. I now comprehend the benefits of the earthen pot, enhancing the water's mineral density. Despite not having a refrigerator in our chawl house, the water from the matka always delivered a refreshing and cool taste, especially after enduring long runs and games during scorching summers.

'Beta, sit down first. Don't drink the chilled water immediately,' I fondly recalled my mother's repeated advice. 'Relax, cool down, and then drink.' Now, modern science reaffirms the wisdom of ancient practices—sitting down before consuming water is essential. Furthermore, the body absorbs cool water more effectively.

During those formative years, my mother predominantly cooked using copper utensils. As a nutritionist, I now comprehend the significance of copper as a metal that purifies bacteria and preserves nutritional value. We also enjoyed our meals on clay plates, embracing the healthful tradition of earthenware.

Mealtime adhered to a well-regulated schedule as we grew up. The children were expected to be home by 7 p.m., and my father would return by that time as well. We had half an hour to freshen up before gathering around my mother's beautifully embroidered bedspread for dinner, which was served promptly at 7.30 p.m.

Of course, the meals themselves were a tantalising blend of health and flavour. We delighted in the spicy coconut curries brimming with potatoes, vegetables and chicken. As a child, I initially only consumed curry and potatoes, being fussy about the meat. However, my mother insisted on my protein intake, and over time, I grew to appreciate its benefits. This protein consumption now aided my recovery, facilitating the development of stamina and muscle.

The fact that I was never a fussy eater, always willing to savour whatever was served, made my life considerably easier during this preparatory period as well.

First Marathon Training Sessions Begin

Compared to cycling, running proved to be a high-impact exercise, necessitating a better diet and increased muscle strength. However, I had to be cautious since running outdoors was off-limits. The treadmill became my sole option.

I approached the gym staff, requesting them to thoroughly disinfect the treadmill before I began my sessions. I started with a slow shuffle, gradually progressing to a slow run. It was challenging, considering the weight gain caused by the steroids and immune suppressants. While cycling allowed for a seated position, shedding pounds via running required a different approach. 'Start by embracing clean eating,' I jotted down in my planner, 'Weight loss will naturally follow.'

* * *

My passion for food and fitness traces back to my college days when I first grasped the significance of eating clean. Any kind of sport held a special place in my heart, and I aspired to build a career around it. Firoz did suggest typewriting classes, but I simply wasn't interested. That's when he accompanied me to a vocational guidance counsellor, a talk with whom revealed that my top career choices were sports, followed by agriculture, and lastly, cooking.

At the time, we couldn't fully comprehend this analysis, and my family suggested I opt for a Bachelor of Commerce degree at the nearby Shrinivas Bagarka College in J.B. Nagar. It was a strategic decision, as it allowed me to continue pursuing sports at the Andheri Sports Complex while also working as a martial arts trainer. My master had offered me a job training school girls in Kung Fu at the Divine Child Girls' High School. Bagarka College was an ideal fit since it was within walking distance of all my training sessions, and the timings aligned perfectly with my schedule—I trained in the morning before college, and resumed my training in the evening, after college.

When I was in 12th grade, I came to realise that my knowledge of nutrition was lacking. During martial arts competitions, I would often feel exhausted after the initial four or five rounds, losing focus in the process. I wondered if it had anything to do with my diet. Determined to enhance my understanding, I sought out colleges that could provide nutrition training.

I discovered that a degree in hotel management would educate me not only on nutrition, food science and hygiene but also allow me to explore the world of culinary arts. My vocational tests further affirmed cooking is a viable career choice for me. However, I was determined not to spend three years pursuing this course. After an extensive search, I set my sights on Sophia Polytechnic's one-year diploma programme and eagerly enrolled.

For the first time in my life, studying became an enjoyable experience, and the year whizzed by, filled with productivity and happiness.

Body-building Beckons

In 1995, we relocated to Kalyan. I had given up running and gained weight. But the body-building bug had bitten me, and I was determined to pursue it. I found a coach, Raj Kshatriya, who helped me shed those extra pounds.

To improve my physique, I needed supplements, but money was tight. Firoz, now a mechanical engineer, had more responsibilities with our extended family. There were my parents, his wife Meher, and their two kids, Abraar and Aaisha, along with me.

To fund my body-building aspirations, I took on a sales job at Eureka Forbes, selling water purifiers. Despite the challenges, I managed to sell twelve purifiers. However, I soon realised that Sales wasn't my calling. I also took up a job as a gym attendant in Kalyan, ensuring I could use the gym for my workouts. In the meantime, I completed my hotel administration course and earned my certification.

In my quest for a sculpted physique, I experimented with both supplements and steroids. They helped me participate in competitions at the district level in Kalyan, occasionally competing in the categories of 'Strong Man' and 'Endurance Man'. However, my coach, a wise man, advised against using steroids, especially the banned anabolic ones, which were often misused to enhance performance. They were addictive and increased my craving for more. They pumped up my body and made me feel powerful. Yet, my coach knew better and strictly prohibited their use.

As a professional bodybuilder at the Thane district level, I didn't agree with the idea of relying on chemicals to shape my physique. It wasn't the right approach for achieving true health and fitness. After a few years and competitions, I decided to step away from professional bodybuilding due to my aversion to consuming a multitude of chemicals.

My experience with steroidal cancer treatment further solidified my resolve to adopt a clean and natural approach to nutrition. I had done it before, and I was ready to do it again.

Now, I was gearing up to run my first-ever marathon. It was October, and the scorching Mumbai heat was stifling.

As always, I devised a schedule: two runs a week, two cycling sessions a week, and daily 20-minute strength training sessions, followed by breathing exercises and meditation. I also incorporated stretches to improve flexibility. The commitment to food hygiene, with sterilised and steam-cooked meals, remained a priority.

By December, I was gradually regaining my former self. It took two months of consistent effort to run five kilometres without a break. It might not have been a great distance, but the feeling was incredible.

18

FIRST FLAG-OFF!

January 2015 arrived, marking the beginning of my preparations for the Comrades qualification. Dhananjay Sandu, the managing director of Tridhaatu Realty and Infra Pvt. Ltd, and a Virtus client, was organising the Chembur Monsoon Marathon in August 2015. This 10-kilometre run seemed like the perfect opportunity to assess my endurance levels. Despite being in the initial two-year window period following my bone marrow transplant, which Dr Bhave emphasised as the 'most crucial years' during every check-up, I enrolled for the race.

Time flew, and before I knew it, six months had passed. I participated in my first 10-kilometre run, completing it in an exhilarating 53 minutes. The sense of achievement fuelled my determination to take on the next challenge: completing the 21-kilometre half marathon at the Standard Chartered Mumbai Marathon in January 2016 under two hours.

Even though I faced ongoing health issues, I managed to run non-stop for 18 kilometres by Christmas. I took every precaution necessary to avoid infections that could potentially hinder my participation in the upcoming marathon. Finally, the time had come to put myself to the test in a longer run.

17 January 2016. Mumbai came alive with festivity on marathon day, transforming its typically laid-back fitness attitude for that one morning. With 44,000 participants warming up, the atmosphere was electrifying. Professional runners and amateurs, all gathered with various motivations—raising funds for social causes, seeking entertainment, or simply cheering on the runners. Mumbai's vibrant energy contrasts the quiet and peacefulness of Pune, and I revel in its pulsating spirit.

Nitin, who had registered for the full 42-kilometre marathon, and I arrived at the starting point at 5.15 a.m. The race commenced half an hour later, and off we went, joining the massive crowd of 44,000 runners.

At the halfway mark, I recalled my promise to Jesal Shah, one of Virtus's members, that I would pace her during the second half of the marathon. Jesal, who had been training under Nitin, was running her first half-marathon, and I was determined to help her achieve her personal best. After all, as the Comrades emphasises, marathons are about celebrating teamwork, camaraderie and supporting one another.

The locals, even those not participating, had gathered early on a Sunday morning to cheer and volunteer. They offered water, lime juice, fruits, juices, cookies, dates and even cakes to strangers. Their selflessness and genuine happiness in assisting the runners were truly remarkable. Encouraged by the crowd's motivation, Jesal and I navigated through challenging stretches of the marathon with ease.

As we approached the finish line, I realised that in my effort to spur Jesal on, I had fallen behind on my own time goal. With her consent, I sprinted towards the finish line and completed the half marathon in 01:59:20 (1 hour, 59 minutes, 20 seconds)! I had done it! Jesal too achieved her personal best with a time of 2 hours and 9 minutes.

The atmosphere and the moral support provided by the Mumbai Marathon inspire participants to return year after year. It's more than just achieving personal bests; it's about embracing the spirit of participation and the sense of community that pervades the event.

Train For the Full Marathon

With 21 kilometres done, it was time to shift gears, double the volume and the distance. That would require even better focus and of course, much more training. But I knew my immune system was not optimum and needed to be worked upon. I had one year to up my game.

I started preparing the next training plan. I wanted to listen to my body and go accordingly. For that, I decided to budget four months for infection-related illnesses and their recovery periods. Experience had taught me to be prepared. That meant I had eight months of preparation time.

I broke up this annual goal into shorter goals and decided to run another half marathon but in more challenging terrain. I researched my options and shortlisted the Nilgiris Ultra Marathon scheduled for November 2016. When I shared this plan with Nitin, he excitedly suggested we plan a short vacation post the marathon.

But we set separate goals. Nitin, who had already run a 42-kilometre marathon, decided to go the ultra-distance and enrolled for the 75-kilometre run. He was confident of completing it. I chose the 25-kilometre one. It was almost the same as the Mumbai half marathon but would be tougher given the hilly terrain with its aggressive climbs and descents.

The Nilgiris in the mountains of Ooty required special training. My Mumbai runs were mostly on flat surfaces. So, Nitin and I had to find a similarly simulated area in Mumbai where we could practise climb training. We zeroed in on Thane's Yeoor Hills which is on the outskirts of Mumbai.

It was February 2016. Before starting the training, I needed to build my body, strengthen my legs and start building a base. It was vital because base-building would include cardiovascular training and running, both required for long-distance running.

To build further endurance, I started slow long-distance runs and used the Dr Phil Maffetone aerobic heart rate zone to control my still-rather-erratic heart rate. I was a 'techie' runner and loved to number crunch. I needed to hit the gym to start strength and conditioning training as well.

I always follow the linear progression method and advise my trainees to do the same and wrote down a three-week timetable followed by a recovery period in week 4 at a reduced volume.

* * *

Three weeks of conditioning and running had passed, and Nitin and I decided to embark on a short test run of five kilometres in the Yeoor Hills. But it served as a sharp reality for me as I could only manage a painfully slow jog.

Although I completed the five-kilometre run, it served as a stark reality check, revealing just how weak I was.

Desperately, I began scribbling again:

- *Need to strengthen my legs.*
- *Focus on improving breathing techniques.*
- *Increase cardiovascular conditioning.*
- *Make it a point to visit Yeoor Hills at least twice a week, gradually increasing the distance each time.*

The Uphill and The Downhill

Nitin and I meticulously devised a comprehensive training plan, methodically working on enhancing our cardio endurance, refining our breathing techniques and diligently conditioning our bodies for the rigorous uphill runs. The initial goal of five kilometres swiftly transformed into a commendable six, and within a few weeks, our determined efforts propelled us to conquer the challenging eight-kilometre mark.

Eager to push our limits, we ambitiously decided to tackle a maximum of ten kilometres in a loop, encompassing the arduous ascent and descent, repeating this demanding pattern for an impressive five loops.

Suffused with a profound sense of satisfaction, I found solace in reminiscing about the captivating allure of the Mumbai Marathon—the enchantment that ignited my passion for racing and the momentum it kindled, which carried me through the subsequent three months of dedicated training.

Surprisingly, within this remarkably brief span, I rapidly and resolutely escalated my mileage, meticulously logging an impressive 52–54 kilometres every week. The fruits of my tireless labour manifested as a tangible achievement—I triumphantly conquered the uphill challenges five consecutive times, unwavering in my stride, while astutely managing the rigorous downhill sections with remarkable efficiency and composure.

Monsoons Brought Infections

Winter had transformed into summer, and the scorching heat didn't faze me until the arrival of the rains. Mumbai's monsoon bestowed vitality and splendour upon the city. The refreshing winds tempered the oppressive warmth and the trees turned green once more. However, for me, it was a contrasting tale as the rains seemed to invite a relentless onslaught of infections.

It started with the flu. This bout of illness prompted Dr Bhave to instruct me to get vaccinated. A viral followed soon enough. The compulsory bed rest and lack of exercise were irritating me. The viral infection had sapped me of my strength, rendering me too feeble to undertake any activities. I was frustrated and desperate to resume normal activities. After all, I had endured over two months of house arrest. My restlessness and discontentment began to wear on my mother's nerves.

'Stop feeling frustrated and redirect your focus,' she reprimanded me sternly one day.

She was right. Determined to resume running within the next 10–15 days, at the very most, I set my sights on the upcoming Satara Hill half-marathon—an arduous run spanning a challenging 10.5 kilometres uphill in the first half.

I yearned to experience it, as it was a shorter version of the Comrades Marathon. However, with the event scheduled for August and mid-July already upon us, I doubted if I would be able to get fit in time. I had to let go of participating in the Satara Marathon. 'Stop moping and look beyond it,' my mother retorted. It buoyed me to hit the gym by mid-August and resume my training regimen.

Despite the recurrent bouts of flu and viral infections, I discovered that my body possessed greater resilience than I had anticipated. Gradually, I incrementally augmented my weekly training workload, steadily increasing the total distance covered. Before long, I achieved a remarkable milestone: for the first time, I surpassed a weekly run volume of 64 kilometres. The sense of achievement was truly exhilarating!

At this juncture, it became imperative for Nitin to increase the distance he ran, aiming for the lofty target of 75 kilometres. It was now my turn to reciprocate the support and assist him in his pursuit, allowing him to concentrate on achieving his objective. Our mutual understanding was so good that we didn't even require explicit communication. We became running companions, training comrades and harboured identical aspirations. Finally, as the week drew to a close, we triumphantly completed a non-stop, long-distance hill run spanning an impressive 20 kilometres.

Karma Comes Around to Itch

Just as things were looking up for me, there was yet another hurdle in store. In the initial week of September, I received a diagnosis of herpes zoster infection. Painful, round, red sores appeared near my waist. Once again, I had to undergo a treatment regimen followed by a fourteen-week maintenance phase. Herpes is notorious for recurring easily in individuals with compromised immune systems. Furthermore, it brought about neuralgia, a persistent tingling sensation that left me restless and unable to engage in running.

Lying at home, my mind wandered back to the mischievous days of my childhood, when I would stumble upon those itching berries up on the rock at Pereirawadi. That discovery became the catalyst for countless pranks I played. Stealthily, I would slip them inside my classmates' shirts and derive great amusement from watching them scratch their backs in bewilderment. On numerous occasions, exasperated parents would storm to our doorstep, complaining to my mother. Eventually, she gave me a stern scolding, issuing an ultimatum for my pranks to cease. And cease they did. Now, I realise the folly of my actions during those times. 'It almost feels as if some higher power is now replaying that childhood joke on me,' I confessed to my mother.

The herpes sores dried up within seven days, but the persistent neuralgia continued to plague me for several days thereafter.

'Always remember your identity. You are a martial artist who thrives on challenges,' I whispered to myself. Over the years, I had engaged in countless conversations with myself, particularly during those frigid nights spent in isolated wards and agonising days filled with relentless pain.

The herpes ordeal had consumed an entire month of my carefully planned schedule. October had arrived, leaving me with just one month until the Nilgiris Ultra Marathon.

Determined, I resumed my training, and after three weeks of intense preparation, the time had finally come to bid farewell to Mumbai and embark on our eagerly anticipated journey to the majestic Nilgiris, nestled high up near Coimbatore.

The Nilgiris Ultra Marathon

10 November 2016. Nitin and I boarded a flight to Coimbatore and then embarked on a scenic cab ride up the breathtaking winding mountain range that cradles Ooty. We were captivated as the towering mountains loomed on our left, while the sheer drop of the deep valley unfolded right outside the cab window.

'This makes our training at Yeoor Hills feel like child's play,' I exclaimed, struggling to catch my breath. Nitin nodded, lost in contemplation about tackling the gruelling 75-kilometre ultra run in such challenging terrain. Fortunately, we had arrived in Ooty two days ahead of the race.

Although Ooty's altitude stands at a modest 1,500 metres above sea level, it would still require some adjustment for us, coming from Mumbai. The crisp, invigorating air infused with the fragrance of swaying eucalyptus trees instilled a sense of optimism. We knew that soon we would acclimatise to the temperature and the higher altitude.

With Thursday evening stretching before us, we decided to take a short walk along the race route. While we had already studied the map, walking the path helped us mentally prepare for the road, the undulating hills and the challenging ascents and descents. Though Nitin exuded confidence, I was aware that my training for the hilly 25 kilometres ahead of me was insufficient. Nevertheless, this realisation did not dampen my excitement or deter my determination in any way.

On Friday, we attended the press briefing and engaged in light exercises, all the while immersing ourselves in the breathtaking beauty of the surrounding mountains.

Race Day

12 November 2016. Nitin's race was scheduled to begin at 2 a.m., with mine following four hours later. Our hotel conveniently stood just two kilometres away from the starting point, so we prepared ourselves to make our way there. We requested a cab post-dinner, but the front desk informed us that no transportation would be available at that late hour.

We chuckled at the situation and didn't let it bother us much. Two kilometres didn't seem like a significant distance. We decided to commence our walk a little past midnight, aiming to reach the start point comfortably. However, we hadn't anticipated the conditions that awaited us as we stepped out of the hotel.

The air was freezing, there was dense fog and it was pitch black all around. The pungent scent of eucalyptus permeated the air. The streets were deserted and visibility was poor. We were ill-prepared for such circumstances.

Concerned, I turned to Nitin and asked, 'How will you manage at 2 a.m. in this darkness?' Fortunately, Nitin was extremely well-prepared. He retrieved a headlight and donned it, which helped us navigate our steps. Nevertheless, the chill gnawed at our bones, and we ran at a decent pace to keep ourselves warm.

As we approached the start line, we noticed only a handful of participants for the 75-kilometre ultra race, and even fewer for the 100-kilometre event, both of which were set to commence at 2 a.m.

'This is nowhere near the festive Mumbai Marathon, is it?' Nitin mused, sparking laughter between us as we treated ourselves to a much-needed cup of delicious local filter coffee. I wished him luck, and when the race began at 2 a.m., he disappeared into the fog.

I decided to walk back to the hotel and rest for a while, as I needed to leave at 5 a.m. to reach my start point at 6. I ordered an early breakfast and settled into bed. At 4.45 a.m., after a quick shower and hastily packing a bag with my racing essentials and water, I stepped outside.

The night wind stung my face. It seemed even darker and colder than it had been a few hours earlier, with no sign of dawn. But to my surprise, there was an auto-rickshaw waiting nearby. The drowsy driver found it amusing that someone wanted to run in such weather. Laughing, he agreed to give me a ride to the starting point. Although the warm-up walk didn't happen, I was grateful for the lift. I could always warm up once I arrived.

First things first: another sip of piping hot black coffee. The 20-minute warm-up felt more enjoyable after the coffee had warmed my insides.

6 a.m.

The race began promptly. There were only 24 other participants, mostly hostel students from Ooty's numerous colleges and a knowledgeable army officer familiar with the race route. I quickly decided to follow their lead, being cautious about my limits.

After three kilometres, we left Ooty town and entered the Nilgiri forest, and that's when the race's character changed. The Nilgiris, named after the tall green eucalyptus trees, enveloped us completely. The environment was enchanting, and the air felt pure. Each breath was refreshing, a stark contrast to the rancid diesel fumes of the city. Instead, the air carried a strong aroma reminiscent of mint candies.

The first half of the race consisted of a gradual downhill slope. I maintained a steady pace as the sun began to rise above the horizon. It was one of the most beautiful sunrises I had ever witnessed. 'No wonder the Nilgiris are called the Blue Mountains,' I whispered to myself.

As the dappled sunlight accompanied me, I reached the halfway mark. The van stationed there offered some food—dates, chocolate, sponge-boiled potatoes and water. Kavita Kanaparthi of Globeracers, the organisers of the run, had done an excellent job.

With the sky awash in a delicate pink hue, I grabbed a few dates and swiftly refilled my water bottle. I didn't want to take a long break and resumed running.

The toughest part of the race, the ascent, lay just ahead. The initial few kilometres were manageable, but after approximately 3.5 kilometres, a steep uphill stretch began.

Based on the maps I had studied, I knew it would be a continuous climb for the next three kilometres. However, the incline felt much longer, seemingly stretching on forever. It significantly slowed down my pace, prompting me to run a bit faster even on the slightest downhill stretches.

I observed the strategies of several other runners—walking or jogging uphill and running downhill. I maintained my pace, slightly slower on the ascent and slightly faster on the descent. Fatigue had settled in; these hills felt never-ending.

After completing another 6.5 kilometres, I reached another hydration point. I opted for half a potato, and two dates, and refilled my bottle once more.

Now, with only six kilometres left, I aimed to increase my pace. The next three kilometres through the forest were swift, and I didn't have time to fully absorb the serenity of the wilderness. Soon, I found myself back in the city for the final three kilometres. I continued running at a brisk pace, grateful for all the training I had pushed myself through, despite the challenges of flu and herpes. The last 200 metres featured another steep climb straight to the finish line, but I didn't falter and maintained my pace.

8.55 a.m.

Crossing the finish line, my time was recorded at 02:55:00 (two hours, 55 minutes). 'Fourth place,' the referee announced.

I was taken aback and pleasantly surprised. I had never imagined that I would achieve fourth place! Furthermore, I had never anticipated how much I would relish this stunning terrain. The run through the forest had been a truly spectacular experience.

Without delay, I stretched after the race and devoured my post-race breakfast. I hopped into a waiting auto-rickshaw and headed back to the hotel. I intended to relax, recover, have lunch, and return before 4 p.m., the cut-off time for Nitin's 75-kilometre run.

4 p.m.

I was overjoyed to witness Nitin crossing the finish line. We embraced and immediately began sharing our race experiences. I assisted him with post-race stretches, feeling like I was repaying a tiny portion of the support he had provided me throughout my cancer journey.

The rickshaw ride back to the hotel was filled with race details, as was our evening snack. As we watched another magnificent sunset over the Nilgiris, a sense of unity with the mountains washed over us—a calm and joyous peace enveloped our beings. With darkness descending, we decided to venture out for dinner. We wanted to celebrate our achievements, our first race outside of Mumbai, and our first ultra-distance. The feeling of conquering both the ups and downs—of the mountains and of life itself—and the sheer pleasure of being alive. We still had two more days to relish in Ooty. Our itineraries awaited us.

Full Marathon: Harder, Faster, Longer

Unlike all those years spent in and out of hospitals, these joyous days of marathon running whizzed by. I returned to Mumbai and promptly fell victim to another bout of the flu. By the time I recommenced my training, it was already December. Now I had a mere 45 days to prepare for my inaugural full marathon, a daunting 42 kilometres, scheduled for 15 January 2017—the Standard Chartered Mumbai Marathon.

Worry consumed me, but my determination remained steadfast. 'I shall undertake this challenge solely to experience the essence of a long-distance run, even if it does not result in a personal best,' I confided to Nitin.

Mumbai's winter posed hurdles to outdoor mileage accumulation. The frigid climate and diminished humidity, coupled with escalated pollution levels, made running outdoors an arduous task. Despite maintaining a low-intensity training regimen, I found myself afflicted with a persistent cold and nagging cough. Although not severe, this setback prevented me from training according to my intentions and plans.

'Gritting my teeth, I shall conquer the marathon,' I resolved silently, with unwavering determination.

19

THE FULL MARATHON

1 January 2017. I was determined to start the year on a high note. My goal was to achieve my longest run yet. I reached my daily running starting point earlier than usual. Even at 3.45 a.m., the Mulund service road was bustling with cars zipping by. Most Mumbaikars were either returning from New Year's Eve parties or heading to another. I dedicated nearly 20 minutes to warm up.

The morning enveloped me with its cold, foggy and dusky atmosphere. The service road did not have streetlights, shrouding the entire lane in darkness. The only sources of illumination were the beams of passing cars and trucks. Usually, Nitin accompanied me during training, equipped with a head torch. However, today I found myself alone. Luckily, I had a small torch with me. With great care, I commenced my run, diligently observing each footstep.

The tranquillity allowed me to discern the resonating thud of my footsteps pounding the pavement. 'This is the finest part of early morning runs,' I smiled, assessing my stride and running mechanics based on the impact of each footfall. The sound of my breath helped me synchronise it with each step. It also brought forth a wide smile as childhood memories of early morning runs came flooding back.

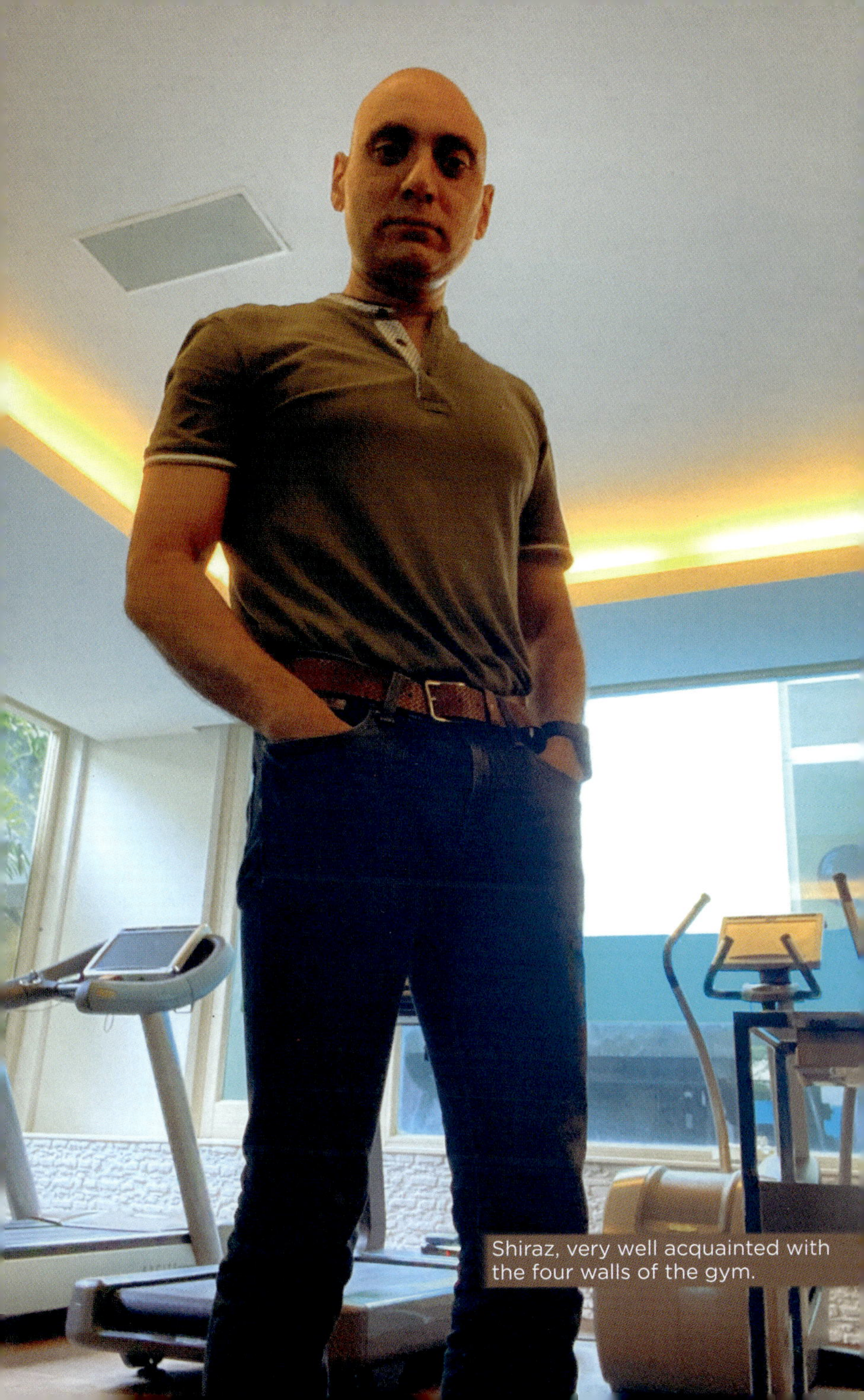

Shiraz, very well acquainted with the four walls of the gym.

Running the Maharashtra Police International Marathon, 9 February 2020.

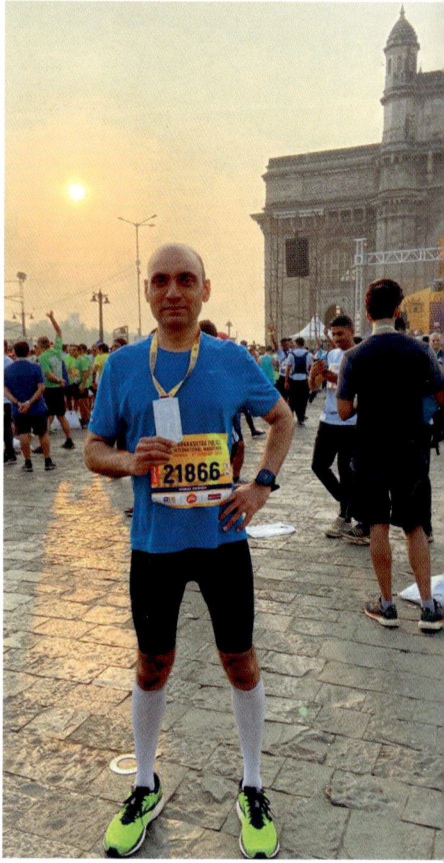

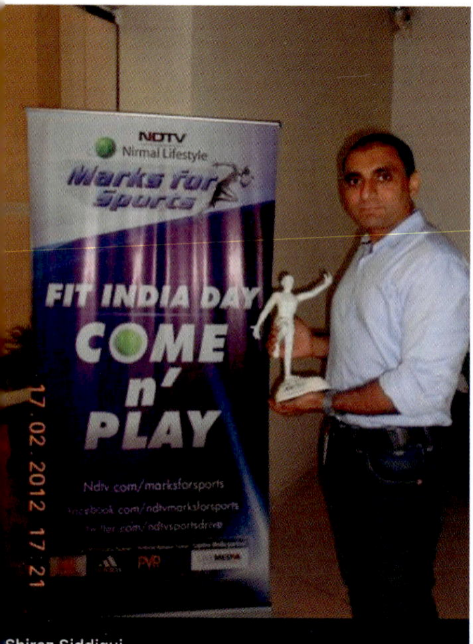

Shiraz felicitated with the prestigious Lifetime Achievement Award for the 'Against the Odds' category in 2012, for his contributions to and association with the 'NDTV-Nirmal Lifestyle Marks for Sports campaign'.

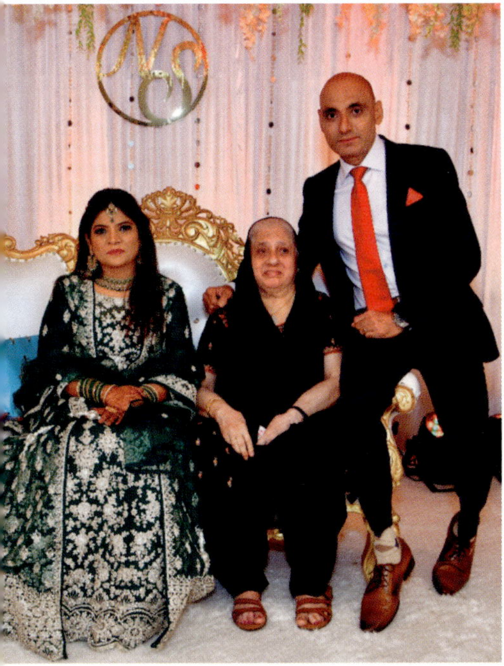

Shiraz on his wedding day, all smiles with his wife Nida and his mother.

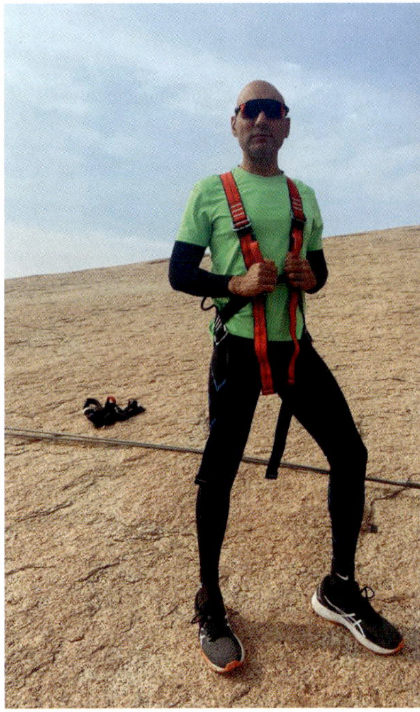

Shiraz during the Rock Climbing Course (Level 1) in Telangana, October 2021.

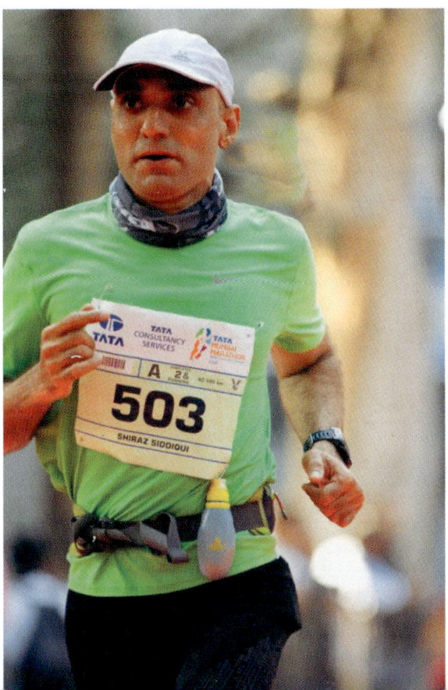

Shiraz, inspiring as ever, running the Tata Mumbai Marathon 2020 for the fourth time.

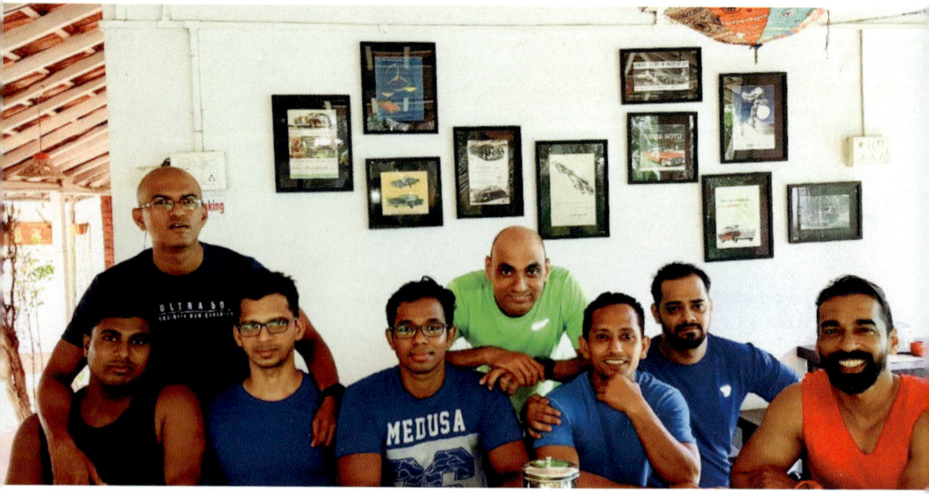

Shiraz with the cheery Virtus group during the trip to Alibaug, May 2019.

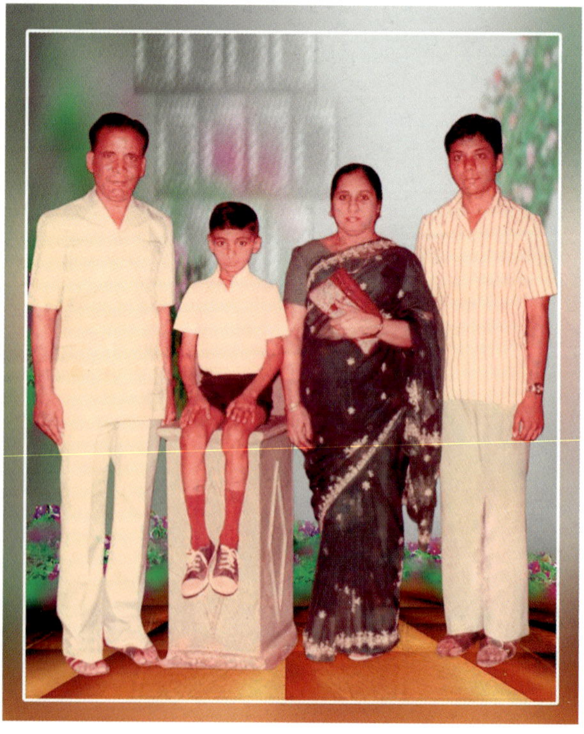

The family — his father, Shiraz, his mother, his brother Firoz — from Shiraz's childhood days.

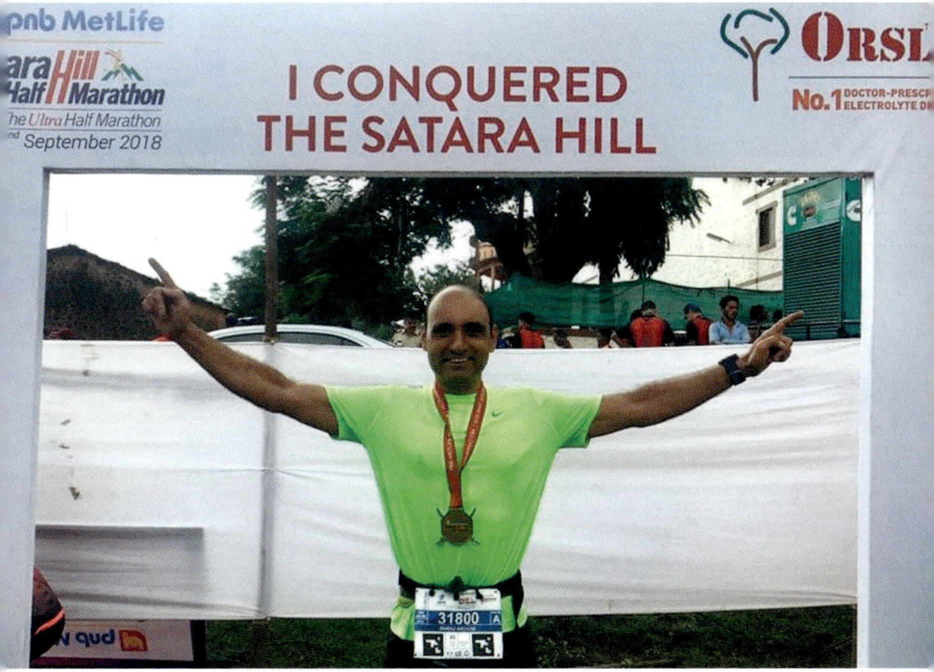

Emerging victorious after the PNB MetLife Satara Hill Half Marathon, 2 September 2018.

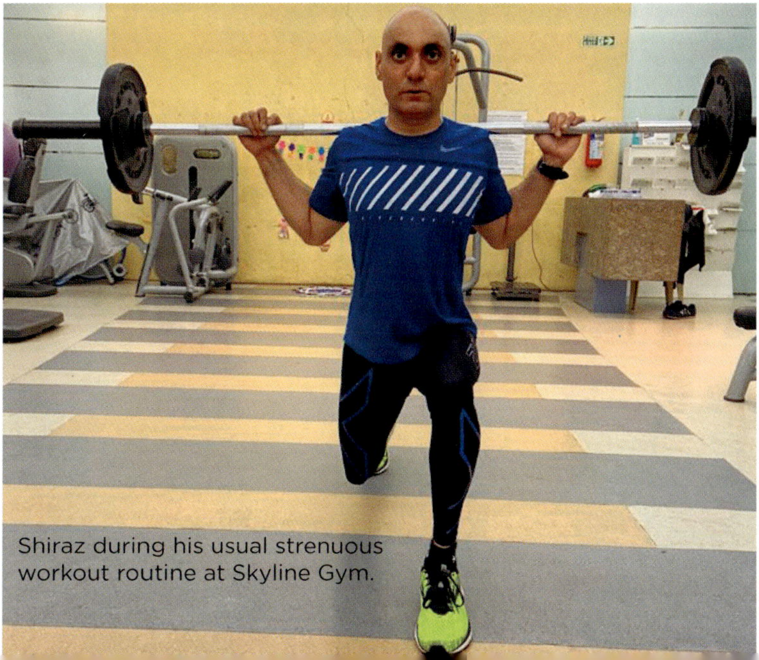

Shiraz during his usual strenuous workout routine at Skyline Gym.

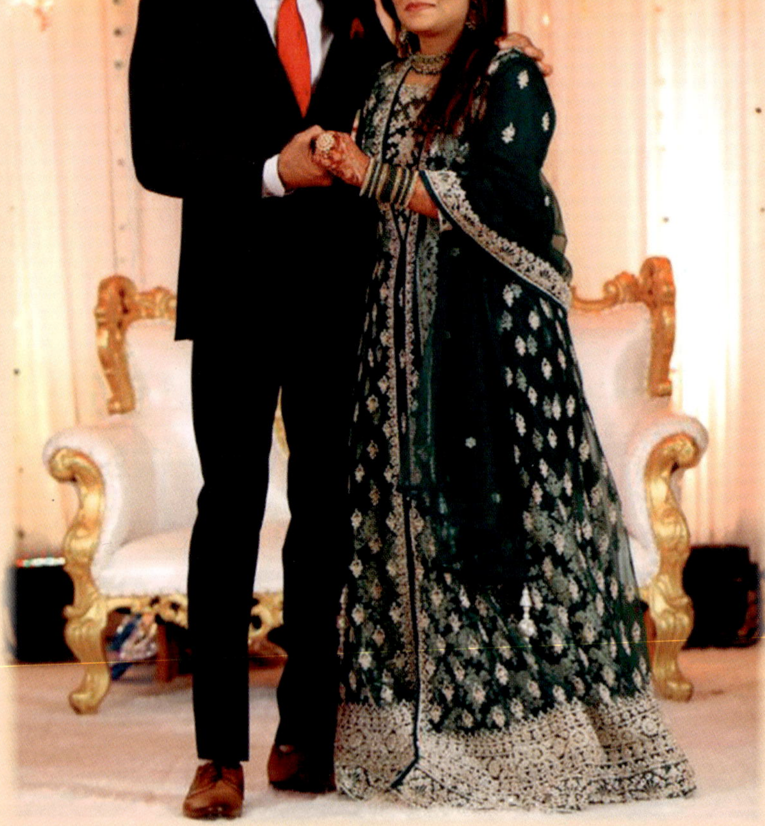

The happy couple during their Walima, the post-wedding celebrations.

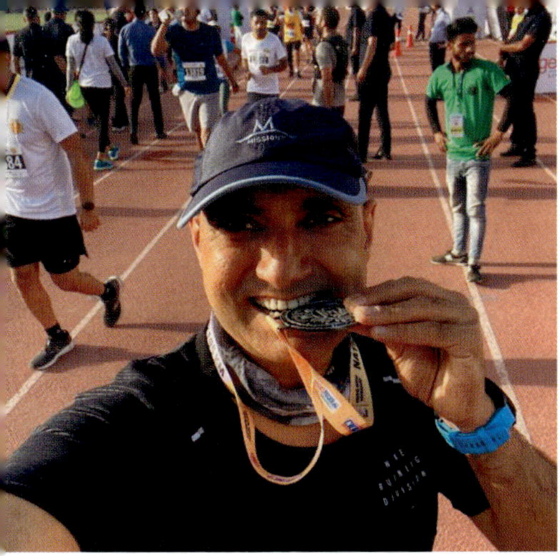

Finishing the amazing Thailand Marathon in Bangkok, his very first international run, 4 February 2018.

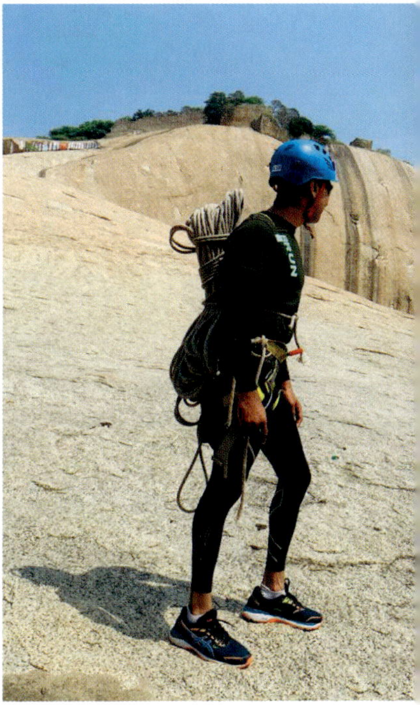

Another still of Shiraz participating in the Rock Climbing Course (Level 1) in Telangana, October 2021.

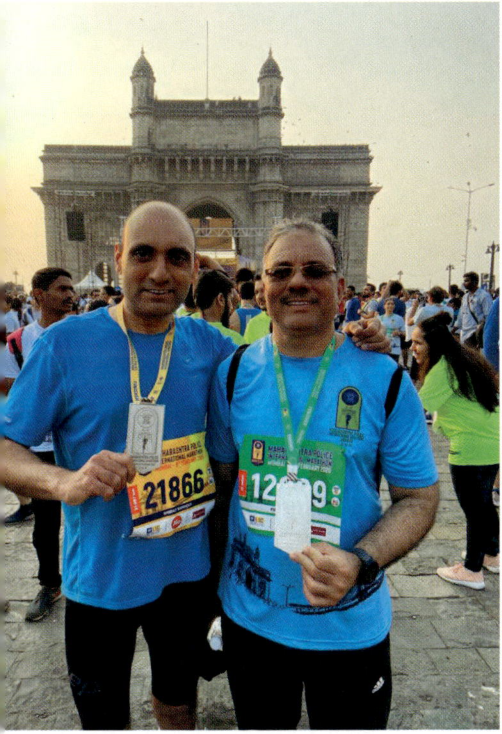

Concluding the Maharashtra Police International Marathon with his brother Firoz Siddiqui beaming by his side, 9 February 2020.

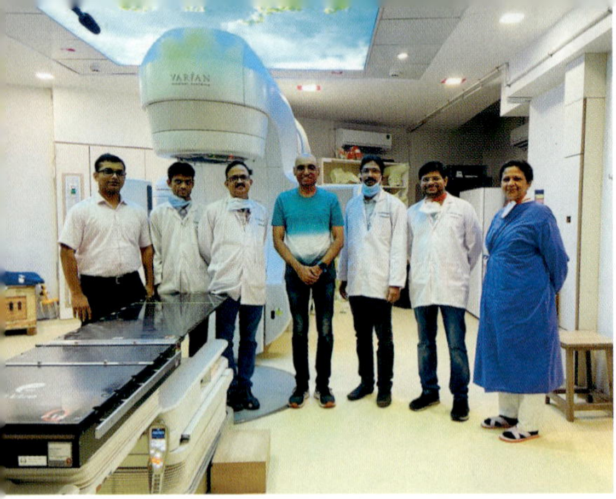

Shiraz on the day of his final radiation treatment in August o 2022, posing with the talented Hinduja Hospital radiology tean in front of the state-of-the-art radiology equipment.

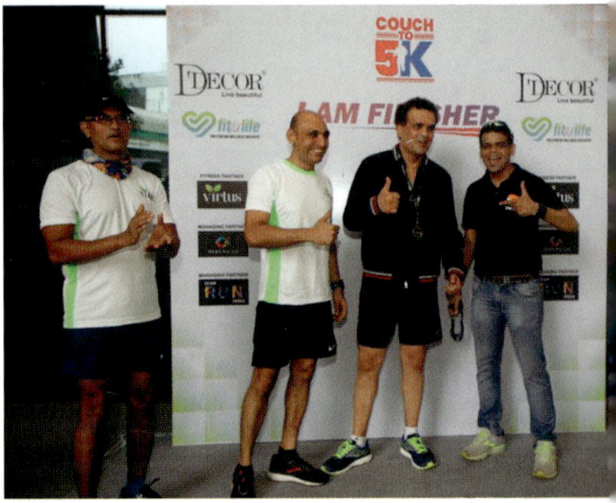

After the Couch to 5k run organised by Virtus for D'Decor, Season 1, October 2019.

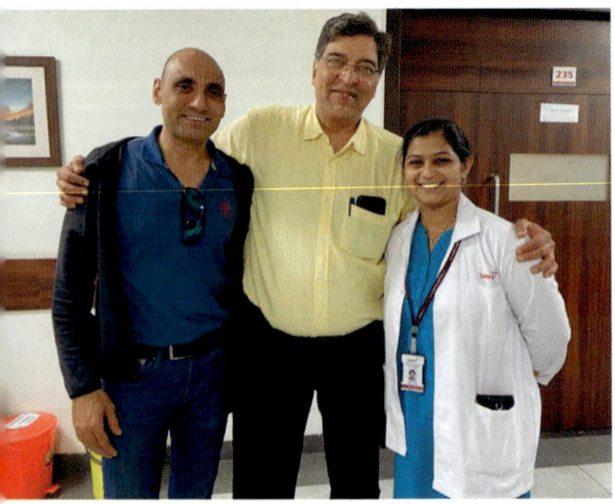

Shiraz standing with the proficient doctors, Dr Shashikant Apte and Dr Aditi, around the time of his Bone Marrow Transplant.

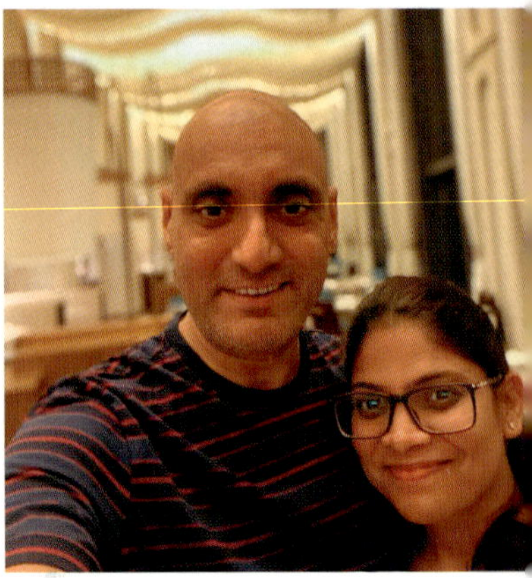

Shiraz posing for a selfie with Nid

'This time, it wasn't just those five kilometres,' I reminded myself. I aimed to accomplish my longest run yet, surpassing the distance of the Mumbai Marathon's 21 kilometres and covering three-quarters of the way towards the full marathon. My target for the day was at least 26 kilometres. The service road stretched nine kilometres in one direction, and I planned to traverse the entire length three times over.

One run was completed, and I executed a U-turn. Soon, I reached my starting point again, having covered 18 kilometres. I felt invigorated.

Once again, I executed a U-turn. It was time for the final segment of the morning. By the time I reached the 21-kilometre mark, having covered another three kilometres, I felt re-energised.

Executing a U-turn from the midpoint allowed me to conclude where I had started. Only 4.5 kilometres remained to achieve my goal for the day. As I ran this stretch, the anterior part of my shin muscles started to throb. It became evident that anterior tibialis muscle fatigue was setting in. Each step seemed to tighten the muscles further as if I were lifting a weighty log instead of a leg.

* * *

I allocated myself a two-day window for complete recovery. I diligently engaged in extensive foam rolling, employing it as a form of self-massage to alleviate the knots in my body and expedite the healing process. With the weekend on the horizon and the imminent Mumbai Marathon drawing closer on 15 January, it was expected that I would gradually reduce the intensity of my training, a technique known as tapering.

However, I deviated from this plan. Having already missed nearly three months of training due to herpes recovery, I was determined to squeeze in one more long-distance run. Nitin and I devised a plan to cover 23 kilometres. This time, we opted for a route that took us from Worli Sea Face to the National Centre for Performing Arts (NCPA) at Nariman Point, before returning to Worli Sea Face.

To my surprise, the run felt considerably more manageable compared to the previous Sunday morning's outing in Mulund. Following a route that closely resembled the Mumbai Marathon's planned race course, it felt like a rehearsal for the actual event.

I completed the run, albeit feeling utterly drained. In the subsequent week, my legs exhibited signs of fatigue. I didn't possess a notable sense of fitness as the race day approached. I hadn't fully recuperated, nor had I effectively tapered down my training.

Nevertheless, I clung to my goal. I was on a mission.

Race Day: The Full Mumbai Marathon

15 January 2017–5.30 a.m. Standing at the start-line of the Standard Chartered Mumbai Marathon held a special significance, even on my second attempt. The desire to run a full marathon had been brewing for a long time. Timing and completion were not my concerns; I felt privileged just to be present. After all, Nitin and I had traversed a long journey as friends, partners and comrades. Contrary to the common belief that the 42-kilometre race is sparsely populated, the initial five kilometres were unexpectedly congested, forcing us to maintain a slow pace.

Soon enough, we immersed ourselves in the race, passing by the iconic landmarks of South Mumbai. The sight of the Arabian Sea, as we began to ascend, was truly awe-inspiring. The grandeur of the Bandra–Worli Sea Link, an integral part of the route, was captivating. The entire course exuded rejuvenation and excitement. As we started descending, Lilavati Hospital came into view, evoking a profound sense of tranquillity. I had triumphed over cancer and was embracing life, leaving behind the distant memories of those isolated days.

At Bandra Reclamation, we made a U-turn on the sea link and reached Mahim, home to the renowned Makhdoom Ali Mahimi Dargah, from which the area takes its name. It made me reflect on the peculiarity of my relationship with religion.

As a young boy, I would evade Namaaz classes and even attempt to slip away during Eid Namaaz. However, when I was grappling with cancer and feeling lost, I hired a tutor to help me read the Quran, not once but thrice. I had sought solace, only to discover that it resided within myself and my passion for running.

I knew my endurance would last only until the 26th- or 28th-kilometre mark. The real test would commence beyond that threshold.

Nitin, on the other hand, had participated in several marathons in different cities and had even completed the ultra-distance at Nilgiris. His fitness and conditioning far surpassed mine.

Precisely at the 29-kilometre mark, my calves began tightening every few metres. By the 33rd kilometre, I eventually had to slow down, walking a few paces. Kind people offered oranges, which I gratefully accepted along with a pinch of salt and 200 ml of bottled water.

I urged Nitin to forge ahead, but he refused, choosing to pace with me. 'It's your first 42 kilometres. We'll do it together. It'll make it more special,' he said with a smile. Once again, I immersed myself in the camaraderie of running.

We resumed running, conquering the climb from the Haji Ali signal, all the way to Jaslok Hospital and my alma mater, Sophia College, at Peddar Road. Drawing from my experience of the previous year, I knew the incline wasn't overly steep. Determined not to walk, I managed to maintain a running stride up the gentle slope.

As the race progressed, my calves throbbed with agony, and I felt completely dehydrated. Despite it being January, typically considered winter in Mumbai, the sun blazed relentlessly, causing the day to be a humid one due to the sweltering heat.

By the time I reached the 36-kilometre mark, I had to pause once more, rehydrate, and walk for the next 500 metres to regain composure. But I refused to halt my running journey after this point. 'The final six kilometres must be conquered,' I gasped to Nitin, who provided unwavering encouragement.

Once again, we embarked on our run, and the finish line loomed in sight. The beckoning red carpet lay just 500 metres ahead. Overwhelmed with exhaustion, I felt as if my legs might give way. However, the resounding cheers from the multitude of spectators propelled me with the surge of adrenaline required to cross the finish line. My clocked time was 04:51:57 (four hours, 51 minutes, 57 seconds). I had finally conquered!

Exhausted yet elated, Nitin and I basked in the glory of the moment. The collective energy of countless positive and like-minded individuals dispelled our weariness. Moreover, the assortment of delectable treats on offer proved invigorating. From cookies to cakes, pastries to fresh fruit juices, smoothies, and even milkshakes—the Mumbai Marathon transformed into a veritable feast of food, culture, and team spirit.

As we awaited the arrival of our colleagues from the team at the finish line, I cherished these moments steeped in the simple joys of merriment, friendship, and yes, even fatigue.

The Accidental Discovery: The Planned Training

'First full marathon completed,' I murmured to myself that evening. 'Now, the goal for the Mumbai Marathon 2018 is to finish the full marathon in under four hours.'

I knew it wouldn't happen effortlessly. Just as I had conquered my mind to complete the 2017 marathon, I would need to master my body as well.

'Like stumbling upon that treasure trove of cricket balls above the Laxmi Narayan temple,' I reminisced, chuckling at the childhood memory. A ladder had been left leaning against the roof by a worker, and the curious kids had decided to scale it, only to be chased away by the construction worker. The ladder swiftly disappeared thereafter.

Yet, what a treasure trove they had discovered—countless kites and a multitude of rubber cricket balls that were deemed beyond saving and left to decay.

When no one had the means to buy a new ball, and this happened at least once a month, I would surreptitiously and skilfully climb the nearest Ashoka tree and rescue a ball for the team.

Of course, I had a lookout on guard duty. 'If you hear anyone, whistle and run as fast as you can.' It was an intensely serious training regime.

'Just like the training I require now to conquer these marathons,' I pondered as I drifted off.

Over the next four months, I persisted with my training despite being struck down by the flu and viral illness as expected. The year whizzed by, and suddenly I found myself with just two and a half months remaining to prepare for the Mumbai Marathon. Unlike the previous year, when I doubted my ability to finish the race, this time I was confident that I would complete it with ease. My target for this year was to finish it within four hours. I needed to build up speed.

The need for speed was ingrained in me. I recalled racing through those early morning runs before school and pushing myself harder while cycling. I even remembered zipping across the neighbourhood on a kiddie two-wheeler scooter, standing and propelling myself with one leg.

This need for speed had got me into trouble. After teaching Vikas how to ride his brand-new BSA SLR bike, we friends decided to ride together. And quickly. As we gained speed, strong headwinds rushed through our ears, and dust stung our eyes.

'Watch out for pebbles and sand ahead. Start slowing down,' Vikas shouted.

But we were too swift. By the time I hit the brakes, we had already skidded onto the pebbles, sliding across the gravel.

Vikas's elbow was bruised and bleeding and his T-shirt was torn. He looked pitiful, but fortunately, he was alright. As for me, a few scrapes and bruises were to be expected.

After that incident, there was no more riding. Vikas's father came to my house that evening, shouting. Even though my cycling training had been going well for the past two weeks, I felt like a failure that night. However, I immensely enjoyed riding that bike. Sadly, I never got the chance to touch it again. The trust between us boys had been shattered.

Now, ironically, I needed to rediscover that speed within me once more. I had to excel in the Mumbai Marathon.

I planned a leisurely trail run at the Sanjay Gandhi National Park. The stifling heat was gradually subsiding. My target was ten kilometres. After warming up, I began at a slow pace. As I reached the three-kilometre mark, a shooting pain surged through my left calf.

That's peculiar, I thought to myself. I had been training diligently and expected 10 kilometres to be a breeze. I stopped, stretched, took a brief walk, and attempted to run again. However, the pain persisted. Determined to complete the distance, I walked the remainder of the ten kilometres. Yet, after walking merely 500 metres, the shooting pain returned.

I visited the doctor later, who diagnosed it as a Grade I calf strain. I had always been aware of my low foot arch. Now, the physiotherapist confirmed that I needed to strengthen my calves and foot muscles. They advised regular calf stretching to improve flexibility and the use of a heel raise or orthotic heel support to relieve pressure on the calves.

'No running for at least ten days. Then, gradually resume,' the doctor instructed. 'Continue strengthening your calves and use the heel raise throughout the day.'

I had no intention of wasting ten days without any training. Instead, I spent that time cross-training on the elliptical machine, indoor rowing, and later, indoor cycling.

The 10 days dragged on.

Determined, I resumed my running on the 11th day, starting with two kilometres and gradually increasing to five kilometres by the third week of November. The calf pain had vanished, but I had lost a valuable three weeks.

Thankfully, luck was on my side, and I could continue training throughout December—a combination of high-intensity runs, slow long-distance runs followed by speed training. I completed my final long run in the first week of January—36 kilometres—slightly slower than the intended race pace.

By that point, I felt confident and shared my sentiments with Nitin. He, too, felt much stronger and more prepared than the previous year.

* * *

Third Time Mumbai: Tata Mumbai Marathon 2018

21 January 2018. Once again, Nitin and I found ourselves at the starting point of the Mumbai Marathon. This marked my second full marathon, and I felt incredibly fortunate to be able to stand among the world's fittest individuals. The Mumbai Marathon garnered international attention, attracting numerous athletes.

The realisation of still being alive, despite everything I had endured, overwhelmed me. The memories of sitting on the balcony of Lilavati Hospital, dressed in blue-checked hospital garments and wearing a mask, undergoing various procedures, remained vivid. Nitin, observing me, smiled and understood the depth of my emotions. 'Thank you, God,' I whispered to myself.

The sound of the flag-off echoed, and instinctively, my feet propelled me forward as I hit the road.

The familiar sense of euphoria enveloped me, accompanied by the captivating live music played by a splendid military band. Nitin and I ran strategically, ensuring we paced ourselves wisely. We were so attuned to each other that we didn't need to exchange any signals.

I had nearly completed 29 kilometres, and the marathon had progressed favourably for me. Though a painful blister was hampering my speed, I managed to cross the finish line clocking 04:01:00. Annoyingly, I had missed my goal by a mere minute due to that blister.

Nonetheless, I felt elated, as my timing represented a significant improvement of 51 minutes from the previous year. It was an extraordinary achievement to complete the 42 kilometres. Nitin arrived at 04:10:00, delayed by a knee ache that cost him 10 minutes.

I felt incredible knowing that I had joined the ranks of those marathoners who completed a full marathon in under four hours. Of course, I was aware of missing my goal by a minute. That one-minute delay served as ample motivation to push even harder in the Mumbai Marathon 2019. For now, it was time to await the other Virtus runners and relish the moment.

The Mumbai Marathon 2018 saw 680 individuals trained and assisted by Virtus cross the finish line! That, in itself, was a tremendous triumph.

As we laughed and gathered for a photo shoot, my mind drifted back to when I had established Virtus back in 2010, amidst my cancer journey. Dr Bhave had labelled it a 'fitness empire'. Life felt victorious.

20

'I HAVE CONQUERED'

I felt a sense of elation in my life. 'I don't think I've been this happy since Class 10,' I jokingly remarked to my mother. Ammi inquired, 'Did you mean after passing your S.S.C. board exam?' Ammi asked, her eyebrow raised. Laughing, I responded, appreciating how typical it was for my mother to assume my happiness revolved around academics. 'No, Ammi,' I clarified, 'it was the day I became the sports captain of my school and was entrusted with organising the entire P.T. class.'

Ammi nodded, her gaze fixed on the newspaper she was reading, evidently unmoved by her son's naive perspective. How typical of him to believe that being a sports captain was the happiest thing to have happened to him! Couldn't he recognise that he should have been happiest when he emerged from the ordeal of a bone marrow survival? Unable to resist, she posed the question, 'Aren't you thrilled to be free of cancer now?'

I failed to grasp the subtle sarcasm embedded in Ammi's words. 'Of course, thank God I can run again,' I replied.

'That's all he can think about. A hopeless case,' Ammi sighed, shaking her head. She adjusted her glasses and immersed herself in the newspaper once more.

I sat on the couch, a smile lingering on my face as I relished the memories. During Class X, Warke Sir stated, 'Boys should be capable of doing a minimum of 25 push-ups.' Having practised martial arts since Class VII, I was already performing sets of 250, ranging up to 1,000 consecutive knuckle push-ups.

Approaching Warke Sir, I quipped, 'What if I surpass 25? Will I receive an A+++ grade?'

'First,' the sceptical teacher demanded, 'demonstrate how many you can do.'

And so I began.

25. 50. 75. 100. 105.

'Stop. That's more than enough,' declared Warke Sir. Respect now permeated his tone. 'You have performed admirably. I appoint you as the sports captain. You can oversee the entire P.T. class and determine the strength, flexibility, and conditioning during the drills.'

It had felt like an incredible accomplishment.

When the bell rang, Warke Sir inquired, 'How did you achieve this?'

'I have been studying Kung Fu since Class VII. I am already in my fourth year of martial arts training. I compete at the State level, I proudly replied, unconsciously standing a little taller. Now the entire school would learn that they harboured a champion in their midst. It was enjoyable back then, and it continues to be enjoyable now.

'I yearn for freedom, to relish life, to be independent and pursue everything I've ever desired,' I murmured sleepily, rising to make my way to the bedroom. 'Tomorrow, I will set new goals for myself.'

Fourteen Years of Endurance

The Comrades Marathon consumed my thoughts, its significance resonating deeply with my personal journey. My battle against cancer had endured for approximately fourteen years. The Comrades, much like my fight, represented endurance and triumph over apartheid, a social disease. Over the past fourteen years, I had confronted life's challenges head-on and emerged victorious. Every treatment and protocol, whether it involved a huge load of antibiotics or a daunting transplant, I accepted, acted upon, and followed.

Certainly, some obstacles shattered my body and spirit. In these fourteen years, I had come face to face with death. Most of my fellow patients I knew had succumbed, not only due to infections but also because they couldn't endure the prolonged years of chemotherapy. It is cancer's relapse that claims lives, breaking people mentally more than physically.

In the Comrades, I envisioned a race that tested endurance in the same vein. It felt deeply personal. I would participate not for the ultra-distance itself, but to pay homage to the mental resilience required to combat cancer.

And along the way, I would honour my angels. The spirit of the Comrades, steeped in African ubuntu, embodied camaraderie. Similarly, I had experienced assistance and kindness from individuals I barely knew—fellow gym members whom I encountered for only an hour each week, who had provided financial support. Doctors guided me through it all. And, of course, my family—especially my brother, without whom I would not be alive—and friends who became my chosen family. The

Comrades would serve as my way of expressing, 'Thank you for believing in me.'

Back in 2004, when I received a diagnosis of Acute Lymphoblastic Leukaemia (A.L.L.), Dr Bhave had warned me during our initial meeting that my cancer might relapse, possibly necessitating a bone marrow transplant. At that time, those words held little meaning for me as a successful fitness coach. I had believed I could conquer the cancer within a year. How naive I was.

Little did I know that cancer would relapse not once, but twice, draining me physically, socially, emotionally, and financially over fourteen arduous years.

Today, I discerned the parallels between running the ultra-distance marathon and my relentless fight against cancer over those torturous fourteen years. 'That's why I am determined to run the Comrades,' I mused, finishing the last of my breakfast.

Now that I had articulated these thoughts, I felt more inspired than ever before. The race beckoned to me, igniting a resolute drive within.

I had witnessed my body deteriorate to the point where even moving from bed to the washroom seemed an insurmountable task. I had experienced helplessness at its peak. However, I had yet to explore the boundaries of my inner strength.

I decided to participate in the 2020 Comrades. Nitin also expressed his desire to join. This race necessitated special training. Not only did it encompass the gruelling 90-kilometre ultra-distance, but it also traversed treacherous hilly terrain. Furthermore, speed played a crucial role in this race. Strict intermittent markers punctuated the course, and athletes had to reach five cut-off points within a specified time to complete the race. Failure to make it in time to Point A would prohibit progress to Point B. Athletes had been disqualified even if they had a foot in the air over the line marker when the whistle blew.

Excitement coursed through me as I reflected on my progress. My body had undoubtedly grown stronger, my endurance had improved, and my immune system had become more healthier. The time had come to push my endurance further. I eagerly anticipated the training ahead.

'Sḥiraz, amidst all this Comrades talk, I completely forgot,' Nitin interjected, interrupting my train of thought. 'Look at these. Shall we go?'

He handed me advertisements for the Amazing Thailand Marathon in Bangkok, taking place within the next three weeks, during the first week of February.

'Agreed,' I nodded, 'It could serve as a brief but well-deserved vacation.'

'Well then, let's book our flights and hotels,' Nitin smiled, retrieving his phone and getting down to business.

The Amazing Thailand Marathon Bangkok

Nitin and I arrived in Bangkok the day before the marathon, brimming with enthusiasm like two young vacationers. We had registered for the 21-kilometre half-marathon, aiming to prioritise our trip as a holiday while staying active.

True to our routine, we utilised our free evening to explore the city on foot and familiarise ourselves with the race route. It proved to be a delightful experience. The route took us across numerous flyovers and meandered through picturesque landmarks such as pagodas and temples. The arrangements made for the event were commendable.

4 February 2018. It marked our inaugural international marathon, and as we began our run, we were astounded by the meticulousness of the preparations. Every detail regarding the safety, security, and convenience of the participants had been carefully attended to. The entire race route was safeguarded by police officers and the army, while volunteers and doctors accompanied the runners on foot or bicycles, equipped with automatic external defibrillators for emergencies. Even the distances between water stations were indicated along the course.

'Can you sense another stark contrast?' Nitin quipped. 'No potholes in sight!' We burst into laughter and carried on.

Neither of us had set a specific time goal. Instead, we relished the vibrant atmosphere and the exemplary professionalism on display. Surprisingly, we crossed the finish line quicker than anticipated.

01:54:18.

Completing a half-marathon in one hour and fifty-four minutes was a commendable achievement. Satisfied with our performance, it was now time to revel in our vacation plans. We had curated an exciting itinerary, including snorkelling in the pristine waters of Phi Phi Islands, kayaking at the renowned James Bond Island, and immersing ourselves in the bustling street markets. And, of course, indulging in the delectable street food.

With my improved immunity, I savoured the culinary delights without hesitation, sampling as many dishes as possible while remaining cautious. Unlike in India, where street food often poses hygiene concerns, here it was handled with great care—from sourcing fresh ingredients from vendors to proper storage and cooking practices. We enthusiastically dug into the local delicacies, particularly my favourites: steamed rice with mango and pad Thai noodles.

Regrettably, our memorable Thai adventure concluded all too swiftly, but it was an experience we thoroughly relished.

12 Days to B.N.P. Ultra

Upon our return from Thailand, we wasted no time and immediately resumed our training. We signed up for another ultra-distance marathon scheduled for 24 February 2018. Despite the two-week window, we felt adequately prepared given our current fitness levels.

The B.N.P. Ultra, spanning 50 kilometres, was in its third edition and set amidst my preferred location in Mumbai—the Sanjay Gandhi National Park at Borivali.

With the recent completion of the full Mumbai marathon and the Thailand half marathons, I felt physically fit. However, the B.N.P. Ultra presented a fresh challenge—to pace ourselves and enhance our endurance. Nitin and I intensified our training over the next two weeks, considering it a valuable opportunity to gauge our fitness levels.

24 February 2018. Race day arrived, and I arrived at the National Park gate by 5 a.m. Surprisingly, the event boasted only 500 participants, with a mere 84 individuals waiting to run the full 50 kilometres. The remaining participants were divided between the 25-kilometre and 12.5-kilometre races.

'Given the absence of cars in the National Park and the limited number of participants, the race track promises to be even more picturesque than anticipated,' I commented to Nitin.

The terrain was undulating, abundant with lush foliage.

'It may not be as grand as the Nilgiris, but for Mumbai, it exudes an unusual tranquillity,' Nitin agreed. Unlike other marathons, there was no blaring music; in fact, there was no music at all—only the melodious chirping of birds. The absence of crowds meant no boisterous cheers or Zumba dancers. The Sanjay Gandhi National Park adheres to silence regulations, strictly enforced throughout the race.

The race coordinator guided us through the warm-up routine, and at 6 a.m., the race commenced. Nitin and I maintained a steady pace, revelling in the serenity and natural beauty of the surroundings.

We completed the first loop in 90 minutes, with each loop spanning approximately 17 kilometres. The course consisted of three loops in total, ascending uphill towards Kanheri, then reaching Gandhi Tekri before returning to Kanheri Caves to conclude a loop. The second loop transpired within the following hour and a half.

Both of us felt robust and at ease as we approached the 42-kilometre mark—the longest distance we had covered. Strangely, at the precise moment I crossed the 42nd kilometre, a sharp hamstring cramp jolted me, necessitating a brief pause to consume some salt. Although I recuperated, I had to reduce my speed. Ultimately, both Nitin and I crossed the finish line at 05:27:30—five hours, 27 minutes, and 30 seconds. Remarkably, I secured fifth place in my age group, a tremendous source of motivation.

The race served as an insightful prelude to the Comrades. 'It was an invaluable learning experience,' I reflected, acknowledging how the heat and humidity impeded our pace. By the time we completed the race, it was already noon, and the scorching sun persisted despite the park's shade.

That night, after dinner, I sat down to record my running diary, ensuring I logged all the lessons learned to successfully conquer the monumental Comrades ultra-marathon.

- *Prioritise sodium intake*
- *Factor in the effects of heat when planning your runs*
- *Acclimatise yourself to running in hot conditions*
- *Train with greater intensity*
- *Increase training volume*

'I'm an Alien'

The B.N.P. Ultra had served as a clear indicator that if I were to participate in the 2020 Comrades, significant improvements were required in my health and training. And that was exactly what I aimed to accomplish. With a two-year timeline ahead, I needed to focus on increasing volume, enduring tougher training sessions, and strengthening my immune system. Despite four years going by since my bone marrow transplant, I still frequently battled colds and coughs, particularly after long runs. Regrettably, this had become a recurring aspect of my life, though I was hesitant to acknowledge it fully.

It was time for my scheduled visit to Dr Apte in Pune. These biannual appointments had become routine, and this time I did not anticipate anything out of the ordinary. Yet, there remained a lingering concern at the back of my mind.

As per usual, I underwent my blood check-up. However, this time, the results astonished and intrigued both me and Dr Apte. My blood group had now transformed to A2 Rh+, an uncommon combination!

This marked the second alteration in my blood group. Initially, my blood group was A+. Within six months of the transplant, it shifted to my brother's blood group, O+. Now, after four years, it had changed once again to A2 Rh+.

'Wow,' I pondered while waiting for Dr Apte. However, underlying my amazement, there was a hint of worry. 'I hope this doesn't indicate any relapse,' I silently fretted.

'It's an unusual blood group,' Dr Apte chuckled, alleviating my concerns.

'In case I require an immediate blood transfusion, what blood group should be considered?' I inquired.

'They would need to determine your blood group at that very moment. Most likely, A+ should suffice,' the doctor replied.

The thought that my blood group was unique stayed with me as I drove back to Mumbai that evening.

'So many incredible things occur within our marvellous bodies without us even realising it,' I mused to myself.

'I hadn't realised I had cancer brewing within me all those years ago. Now, I hardly noticed my blood group changing—not once, but twice,' I laughed, taking in the breathtaking Sahyadri mountain range before me.

I felt an overwhelming sense of awe and gratitude.

'Thank you, God, for everything I possess now. Thank you for everything I have ever had, including the battle with cancer. It has taught me to cherish each moment of my life. Thank you for this extraordinary new lease on life."

Hilly Satara Beckons

Back from Pune, a wave of relief washed over me as I learned all my tests were clear. As I shared the joke about my 'alien blood group' with my mother over dinner, my mind was already racing towards the next challenge.

March had arrived, and I began researching more marathons. The Nilgiris in October didn't quite ignite my excitement, despite their picturesque route. Then, I stumbled upon the one marathon that had eluded me thus far—the P.N.B. Metlife Satara Hill Half Marathon. It was scheduled for 2 September 2018. I had missed it twice before, once due to herpes and another time due to a viral illness that struck a couple of weeks before the event, taking an entire month to recover from. This year, I hoped luck would be on my side. I registered for the half marathon, a gruelling 21-kilometre course set amidst challenging hilly terrain. It would be the perfect preparation for the Comrades.

I decided to immediately start increasing my training volume, beginning in March. The goal was to work towards running 100 kilometres a week—an unprecedented distance for me. I needed a strategy and devised one for myself by allocating the next four months to focus on it.

I progressed well during the summer months, but the monsoons in June forced me to lay low as I caught a viral infection that grounded me for 45 days. I was frustrated yet again for losing 45 days of training.

'But you've become an expert at recovery training,' my mother smiled. Indeed, she had a knack for putting me back on track. Over the years, with countless hospital visits, I learned how to manage medications and their effects. I had also become adept at restarting my training regimen.

With the cold subsiding, I resumed cycling, recognising it as the ideal low-impact exercise and gradually reintroduced running into my routine.

Fortunately, I had already built a solid base before the viral setback, which worked in my favour. Now it was time to focus on speed and hill training.

Once again, Thane's Yeoor Hills proved to be the best training ground in Mumbai.

August and early September whizzed past, and before I knew it, it was time to depart for Satara.

Up the Hill, We Go!

2 September 2018. This time, my friend Nitin and I decided to embark on a four-hour drive from Mumbai to Satara the day before the marathon, just like we always did. The excitement was palpable as we looked forward to participating in our second real hill marathon.

Upon arriving in Satara, we checked into our hotel and made our way to the expo to collect our race bibs. The morning of the marathon was foggy and overcast, adding to the challenge ahead. To make things more interesting, it was a gun start. Each of us was assigned to different categories, and as soon as the gunshot rang out, we took off. The early morning fog had cooled the air, and there was a gentle drizzle that soon subsided.

The Satara Marathon is aptly named the Satara Hill Marathon for a reason. Though it was just a 21-kilometre half marathon, the first half was predominantly uphill, while the second half was downhill. The climb began almost immediately and continued for about 10.5 kilometres. By the time I reached the peak, I was amazed to discover that despite my exhaustion, my body felt strong. Grateful for the training I had put in, I turned around and began the descent. As I turned, I was greeted by the breathtaking view of the valley below. The lush green expanse beneath my feet was mesmerising. The drizzle returned, now slightly heavier. It seemed as if the sky was leaning down to kiss the hills, and the hills responded by reaching up on their toes to touch the clouds above.

The beauty of the surroundings enchanted me. For the first time during a race, I had no desire to continue running. I simply wanted to sit there and marvel at the stunning valley. And so, I did just that, soaking in the moment. I took deep breaths, capturing mental snapshots of the scene.

Despite being aware of the ticking clock, I eventually rose to my feet and quickened my pace. I was running at a remarkable speed, relishing every single step. The breathtaking view tempted me once again to pause and sit down, allowing nature's painting to captivate me. However, I was only a kilometre and a half away from the finish line. I knew there was a slight incline before reaching it. My calves were protesting, and the remaining 750-metre climb proved to be incredibly challenging. Nevertheless, I had no intention of slowing down. Soon enough, I crossed the finish line, completing the race in 01:48:52 (one hour, 49 minutes, and 52 seconds). I secured the 19th position in my age group among 1,722 runners.

People offered their congratulations, impressed by my timing. After stretching, I eagerly awaited Nitin's arrival. He crossed the finish line later, completing the race in two hours and twenty minutes. We embraced each other in celebration.

Up next: Dubai

After the wonderful experience in Thailand, I set my sights on my second international marathon, this time a full one. The Standard Chartered Dubai Marathon was on the horizon. However, I pondered whether I could tackle both the Mumbai and Dubai marathons, considering they were only five days apart, with Dubai scheduled for 25 January 2019. 'Certainly, you can. Reach a new level of fitness and shed some weight,' urged my spirit.

Gradually, I resumed training and controlling my diet and despite regular attacks of the flu, I persisted.

Knowing that the Dubai Marathon would be held on a flat route, I scouted for a suitable, flat road. I discovered one on Airoli's service road and did a trial run there. The 21-kilometre run felt effortless, as did the subsequent 32-kilometre run.

Late that night, I decided to skip the Mumbai Marathon 2019 and booked my tickets for Dubai, with Nitin as my partner, of course.

* * *

We departed from Mumbai on 24 January 2019 on an early morning flight bound for Dubai. Our destination was Jumeira Beach Hotel, where we collected our race bibs. The pre-marathon event surpassed my expectations, boasting lavishness and exceptional organisation. It was every bit as stunning as the photographs had promised. After lunch, we made our way to the hotel near the city centre, strategically located closer to the race route. Instead of succumbing to the temptation of shopping, we opted to explore the area, engage in some stretches, and retire early.

However, sleep didn't come easily for either of us. The Dubai Marathon had a late start, commencing at 7 a.m., which felt 'remarkably late' compared to the 5 a.m. starts we were accustomed to. Moreover, our hotel was just a 10-minute journey away from the starting point.

'It won't be difficult to get a cab here, unlike in the Nilgiris,' Nitin chuckled, alluding to a previous marathon. 'So, let's attempt to get some sleep.'

'The Mumbai Marathon would have been 21 degrees Celsius, whereas here it's around 29 degrees Celsius. The marathon may start late, but the sun rises early,' I observed, noting that by 9 a.m., the heat would intensify.

'Does it concern you?' Nitin inquired.

'No, I'm simply calculating our hydration needs,' I responded.

'It's midnight. Let's get some shut-eye. Even if we can't sleep, let's lie down and relax as we usually do,' suggested the ever-practical Nitin.

I relished this kind of 'shut-eye' as well, as it granted

me the opportunity to mentally envision the entirety of my race route.

25 January 2019. The following morning, we arrived at the race venue at 5.30 a.m. Being a Friday, it was the UAE's weekly day off, and people were out and about, enjoying the day. Similar to the Mumbai Marathon, the atmosphere was a celebratory one, but there was a distinct difference. There were approximately 30,000 participants compared to Mumbai's 55,000-plus, but the crowd seemed incredibly well-managed. There was no jostling, no stepping on toes, and no brushing of elbows.

'The roads are much wider here,' Nitin remarked, 'It makes a difference.'

'And they're perfectly flat, with no potholes,' I added.

Despite the festive environment, music that was being played was soft yet mesmerising.

'Do you notice the absence of honking?' Nitin commented.

I nodded, totally immersing myself in the atmosphere. People of different nationalities had gathered, making it my first full international marathon. I was prepared and warmed up.

The countdown commenced. Gunshot.

'I'll see you at the finish line,' I shouted to Nitin, waving him goodbye.

We each had our goal times in mind.

As I began my pace, I typically kept an eye out for potholes, uneven surfaces and gravel on the road. However, the wide road here meant I could keep my gaze up and ahead, maintaining an optimal running posture.

Quickly, my confidence grew, and I found myself able to maintain good form while looking forward. After completing the first loop, I entered the second one feeling strong and well. When I reached 25 kilometres, I felt the need to hydrate. I had been consuming my gels, filled with carbohydrates, electrolytes and amino acids every seven kilometres to prevent dehydration in the increasing heat.

At the 33rd kilometre, I experienced a severe hamstring cramp, forcing me to slow down. As expected, it was past 9 a.m., and the sun was already blazing overhead. The heat was causing the cramping.

For the next one and a half kilometres, I took shorter strides, stopped at an aid station, and had a bit of salt. I also grabbed a bottle of Gatorade from the Hydration Counter.

From the 37-kilometre mark, I began to pick up my pace once again. I sucked on a chocolate bar I had brought along, as I always felt a drop in sugar levels during the last 10 kilometres of a race.

I was almost there. Only one kilometre remained. The cramping resurfaced, and my right leg calves and hamstrings throbbed painfully. But I had no intention of slowing down. The finish line, marking my first international full marathon, loomed in my mind.

With just 20 metres to go, I decided to finish the race in style. Purposefully, I threw my arms in the air, as if I were the champion of the marathon, emulating the Kenyan runners. Of course, I had a long way to go to reach their level, but the feeling was truly remarkable.

03:38:31 (Three hours, 38 minutes, 31 seconds).

I achieved a personal best and finished 53rd in my age group among 2075 athletes.

It was an incredibly special moment for me. During those days in the hospital, I had never imagined that I would run my fastest full marathon within five years of my bone marrow transplant.

Entering the wonderfully organized recovery tent, I felt pure happiness. Fresh juices, Gatorade, cold towels, ice packs, physiotherapists and masseurs were all available to aid in my post-race recovery and stretching. I strolled around the expansive tent, savouring my Gatorade to rehydrate. Knowing Nitin would arrive shortly, I made my way back to the finish line, eager to capture some photographs of him.

Nitin completed the race in four hours and nine minutes, achieving his personal best time, although he hadn't managed to break the four-hour barrier.

Nonetheless, we were elated to have accomplished what we had set out to do. We came to race and test our abilities, and we passed the test with flying colours. Now, it was time for a well-deserved four-day post-race vacation. We indulged in shopping and feasted to our heart's content. At a popular fried chicken outlet nearby, we ordered two buckets. The lady at the counter seemed slightly puzzled.

'How many of you?' she asked, smiling.

'Just the two of us,' I replied.

'One bucket should suffice,' she suggested.

'No, we'd like two, please,' we replied, grinning.

To her astonishment, we polished off both the buckets of fried chicken.

Back at the hotel, as I freshened up, I gazed at myself in the bathroom mirror. My body appeared fit, and my eyes sparkled.

The Dubai Marathon had been an incredible, particularly meaningful experience. In just seven days, I would mark five years since my bone marrow transplant. From being a newborn in the incubator, writhing in pain and unable to sit up without assistance, here I was, relaxing after completing my first international full marathon.

'This is truly an immense achievement,' I whispered to myself. I called my doctors, and Dr Bhave and Dr Apte were thrilled to hear about my success.

The feeling of gratitude overwhelmed me.

21

A YEAR OF TRAINING FOR THE COMRADES

For the first time, I felt so confident that I wanted to start training for the Comrades from the following day itself, I told Nitin in the cab on the way home in Mumbai.

'Take a break and start the day after,' Nitin suggested.

'I've dreamt of running the Comrades for so long. It's the ultimate human race. Now, I just can't wait to start my actual training,' I replied excitedly.

Nitin nodded, fully aware of my determination.

Unfortunately, my body had other plans. The flu resurfaced and took two weeks to subside, forcing me to rest for a month. However, I used that time to register for the Comrades.

I desired to resume my outdoor hill training since the Comrades is run on the roads of KwaZulu-Natal province, featuring The Big Five set of hills. The race's highest point reached 2,850 feet above sea level.

I chose to train at the Sanjay Gandhi National Park for its hilly terrain. It was already March when I aimed for an inaugural long-distance run of 50 kilometres. I couldn't manage it at first and had to train more, but I finally triumphed. Week after week, I pushed my limits, covering distances of up to 140 kilometres. Despite the scorching heat, with temperatures surpassing 35 degrees Celsius and humidity levels ranging from 70 to 80 per cent, I resolved to endure. 'I must acclimatise myself to this heat,' I reminded myself, persisting through the gruelling training sessions.

By June end, I accomplished a relentless non-stop run spanning 160 kilometres. With a sense of pride, I shared my journey with Ammi, exclaiming, 'Five years ago, in June 2014, I struggled to cover a mere 100 metres in that Pune park. Now, conquering a volume of 160 kilometres poses no difficulty.'

July arrived, and I was invited to spend six days in Turkey with Ajay Arora and his daughter, Adah, the family behind D'Decor. They were trainees of Virtus and wanted to experience the 'Shiraz lifestyle'. They were looking forward to a wellness vacation at their holiday home, and I agreed to join them.

However, just before our trip to Turkey, I fell ill with the flu again thanks to Mumbai's monsoon and its extremely poor air quality that affects athletes training outdoors. The onset of the monsoon in Mumbai always triggered it.

I missed a few days of training. I wanted to arrive in Turkey fit. I knew the air would be clean, and I could easily restart my training at 100 kilometres a week from the moment I landed.

And I was spot on. As soon as I arrived, I could feel the difference in air quality. I dropped my luggage in the room and headed for a run straightaway. The weather was pleasant, the grass was green, and the ocean was sparkling turquoise.

Throughout those six days, even though I was on vacation, I felt the urge to train hard. The weather was so pure, and so was the food. I indulged in platters filled only with fresh fruits for meals. I understood the importance of eating clean, which was difficult back in Mumbai, and I wanted to make the most of it there. It was a wonderful time to practise running non-stop, to the utter amusement and awe of my hosts.

I felt wonderful, as if I had shed a lot of baggage. 'That constant fear of what people thought and felt about me doesn't bother me anymore,' I laughed with my hosts that night. 'I feel lighter. I run faster.'

Upon returning to Mumbai, the remnants of the cough resurfaced, forcing me to take it easy for a couple of weeks. Towards the end of the month, I began building up my volume again and pursued it till the end of December, increasing my volume and capacity despite health hiccups.

Tata Mumbai Marathon 2020

19 January 2020. The Mumbai Marathon 2020 was as special as it had been the previous three times I participated. The atmosphere crackled with excitement, the crowd roared and the city gleamed. This year, twelve of my colleagues from Virtus joined me, and it was wonderful to run alongside them.

The full marathon, which had felt intimidating and gruelling three years ago, now felt comfortable, thanks to the progress I made with my body and training. As I ran on the red carpet, my breathing was steady and the miles passed effortlessly. I completed the 42 kilometres in no time.

03:35:47. A new personal best time! I couldn't have been more thrilled. Not only was I pleased with my timing, but I was also delighted that my body ran smoothly, without any strain or tension. I had truly come a long way.

Maharashtra Police International Marathon

*9 February 2020***.** Firoz had been training with me for the past four months, having returned to Mumbai after his time in the Gulf. I had convinced him to start training through my persistent nagging.

After the announcement of the Maharashtra Police International Marathon following the Mumbai Marathon, I took the liberty of enrolling Firoz without consulting him.

'What? I'm not running a marathon!' Firoz exclaimed, irritated.

'Give it a go. It's just a short 10-mile run,' I encouraged him.

Firoz was furious. 'Ten miles! That's an incredibly long distance!'

'Nitin will pace with you,' I replied calmly, hoping my composed demeanour would inspire my brother. 'Remember how skilled you were in sports when you were in school? You're my inspiration.'

'That was ages ago,' Firoz softened.

'Come on, give it a try. I've already signed you up,' I urged him.

Firoz reluctantly agreed.

As I initially intended to run the half-marathon of 21 kilometres, Nitin was content to pace with Firoz.

01:36:15. Once again, I achieved a personal best time, excelling in the race.

Unfortunately, Firoz fell ill with a cold and cough on race day. Despite being on antibiotics, he decided to run.

'In 2016, two years after my bone-marrow transplant, I completed my first half marathon. I was ranked 189th in my age group. Today, I am ranked 11th,' I enthusiastically shared with Firoz. 'All thanks to you.'

It was a remarkable source of motivation for me. The ranking filled me with energy, affirming my improved fitness level. It also reminded me of how much further I needed to push myself.

'From here, how far will I go? How much will I explore?' I pondered, feeling as excited as a child riding a bicycle for the first time around their building premises.

I was deeply in love with my journey, embracing both the process and the goal. My unwavering belief in my journey fuelled my running and elevated my endurance.

22

COVID STRIKES

'Three months remaining until the Comrades,' I exclaimed enthusiastically to Ammi and Firoz. 'I'll take a week off for recovery and then give it my all.'

However, once again, a viral infection caused a fever that spiked to 102 degrees Farenheit, requiring me to take antibiotics for the next 15 days. It was frustrating because it meant losing the entire month of February. Only March and April were left.

In the first week of March, I started rebuilding my body from scratch. Initially, I could only manage a weekly total of 40 kilometres. Gradually, I increased the volume, incorporating back-to-back training sessions. On Saturday mornings, I ran between 25 and 30 kilometres at a slightly faster pace, followed by 45 to 55 kilometres at a slower pace on Sundays. Running back-to-back helped build stamina for running non-stop for 90 kilometres, which was crucial for the Comrades.

To succeed in the Comrades, both physical and mental fitness were paramount. Athletes had twelve hours to complete the course, with five cut-off points to reach within prescribed times or face disqualification from the race.

At this stage, it was crucial to incorporate long runs, speed work and strength training into my regimen. I alternated regular hill repeats in my weekly training sessions.

By the third week of March, I had regained my fitness. I completed a 70-kilometre-long run in seven hours and 30 minutes, which left me satisfied. However, I still had work to do as it took me five days to recover.

I adjusted my training schedule, adding more to it. Cross-training, particularly cycling, became part of my routine to build additional strength.

'We're approaching April, and I want to achieve my highest weekly volume,' I told Nitin one morning, feeling positive and strong. I aimed to undertake a back-to-back long-distance training session that weekend.

Suddenly, a significant obstacle emerged. The dreaded Covid-19, which had been spreading through China and Europe, had now arrived in India. After an initial scare, the severity of the situation sank in. It was a highly contagious respiratory virus with no known cure, causing widespread fatalities worldwide. The Indian government implemented a complete lockdown, and the World Health Organisation (WHO) declared Covid-19 a pandemic.

The World Has Changed

And so had my routine changed. Despite being unable to go out for exercise, I continued to wake up early. Some deep breathing, meditation, stretches and a special Shiraz breakfast for Mum and me. 'Let's use this time to further develop ourselves,' I told Mum, trying to maintain a positive outlook.

With the world in a new state and uncertain about the future, I developed the habit of scanning the news. It became part of my daily routine to check in with my team members.

'Is everything alright?' I would inquire.

Suddenly, this simple everyday phrase carried a weight of significance.

Prepare lunch, dust the house, clean, mop and do the dishes and laundry. It's an entirely new routine.

'For the first time, I feel like I need the afternoon nap I used to avoid as a boy!' I joked with Mum.

Evenings were dedicated to indoor exercise. The highlight was wearing a mask and climbing the stairs of my fourteen-storey building for a couple of hours. Then, it was time to resume the cooking and cleaning routine for dinner.

Finally, as Mum settled down to watch her television serials, I would either read or call it a night. It had been yet another tiring day.

Lessons from the lockdown: learn to manage the household. Cooking, cleaning, cutting, chopping, repeat! And, of course, the most important lesson—remain calm. Stay composed even when the food you put so much effort into doesn't taste great. Despite being a hotel management student, it didn't mean I enjoyed cooking every single day. For the first time, I gained a newfound appreciation for domestic help. If I wanted to continue enjoying the things I love in life, I had to acknowledge that I relied on the daily support system.

When the finish line was within sight, the run became easier. However, the initial four-week lockdown was extended indefinitely. As March transitioned into April, the virus continued to keep the world confined indoors.

Even as the mutton sizzled in the pan before me, my mind was plagued by a question: would the Comrades be cancelled?

Sure enough, at the end of May, my inbox delivered the news of the cancellation of the race for the year 2020. Since its inception in 1921, the Comrades had been held every single year, except for a break during World War II. The year 2020 would mark only the second exception ever. And it happened to be the year that I had trained for it.

Coincidental, yet significant.

Historic, without a doubt.

'This time, I can run, but the world is not open for running. However, I am alive, and history is unfolding before us.'

Going Online

The mind wandered freely, roaming in the open; the blood was free of cancer. However, this time my hands were trapped in sticky dough, once again attempting to make edible rotis.

Two hours a day spent solely climbing stairs did nothing for my body or soul. I needed to incorporate more exercise into my routine. I had to adapt and change with the times—once again. I found myself confined, isolated, not something new, not something unfamiliar. This time, however, the whole world was also wearing masks.

The fitness and travel industries suffered the most significant blow. Companies fought to survive. Changes had to be made. The world had to transition online.

In just over a month, Virtus Wellness seamlessly shifted into the virtual realm. The entire team operated online. Online consultations were streamlined. Unlike ever before, people sought fitness resources—not just exercises, but overall health and wellness guidance.

'Is it out of fear or newfound free time?' I pondered with my team.

'Either way, it benefits us,' the team replied.

Virtus launched a virtual personal study programme.

Like everyone else, we adapted.

However, something was missing—my outdoor evening training, my breath of fresh air. The stairs remained faithful companions, but my body yearned for a greater challenge.

'Planks,' I declared.

'I've never been fond of stationary exercises,' I mused, shrugging. 'Even sitting in one place and meditating was quite a challenge. But I learned.'

Yes, planks. My longest plank hold was a mere three minutes.

'I will do it,' I resolved. 'I will work on my planks.'

As the month progressed, my endurance improved. The first 20 minutes were easy. Then, my elbows began to ache. My shoulders, my back, even my toes—everything hurt. But I persevered.

In just one month, the three-minute hold extended to 60 minutes. I marvelled at how this simple exercise could profoundly challenge me, both physically and mentally.

It reaffirmed the lessons my cancer treatment had taught me. The strength to push forward, and the resilience to never give up—these qualities will guide you through.

As Diwali 2020 and New Year 2021 passed by, there were no celebrations. For an athlete, a celebration meant going for a long run. I sorely missed my long runs. But I also felt grateful for the short ones, breathing in the open air again.

The year 2020 was a sprint. Short bursts of fresh air.

23

WEDDING BELLS

If 2020 had felt like a sprint, 2021 turned out to be the ultimate marathon life had to offer. On 15 December 2020, the glimmer of hope that had emerged was ready to blossom into a blazing fire.

In 2020, I reached the milestone of being cancer-free for seven years. It also marked three decades of my mother persistently urging me to get married. However, during the three months of complete lockdown that Ammi and I spent together, my mother had a mission. Mission Marriage. Not a single 12-hour period went by without her mentioning it! Ammi was determined to see me settled!

Eventually, I gave in—partly to bring peace to her relentless pleas, and partly because I didn't expect much, considering my medical history.

'Shiraz has finally agreed to meet potential matches,' the news spread rapidly. My brother Firoz joined forces with Ammi and enlisted the help of a family matchmaker. As one of Ammi's birthday gifts, I had an initial conversation with my future mother-in-law. During that very first phone call (which I hoped would also be the last), I made everything explicitly clear—my past, and my medical background. Surprisingly, she seemed unfazed by it.

'Speak to Nida. If she's happy, we're happy.'

Nida was working in Dubai for a telecom company as a verification analyst and lived with her elder sister's family. On 17 December, setting aside my awkwardness, I finally initiated the video call. To my utter astonishment, I found myself at ease while speaking to this unfamiliar girl.

We discussed our families, routines, likes and dislikes. She displayed genuine curiosity about me, attentively listening to every detail. Likewise, I found her remarkably similar to me. Within minutes of the conversation, she made me feel completely comfortable. I was so at ease that I even dared to ask her about her weight on this very first call!

The conversation flowed effortlessly. Two hours slipped away. I had called at 5.30 p.m. Indian time, and before I knew it, it was 7.30 p.m. Time for her to return to work in the UAE.

'I had expected us to feel awkward and struggle to find things to talk about,' I confessed to Ammi. 'But it felt like talking to a friend.'

Ammi beamed with delight.

However, I needed to proceed with caution.

'We haven't made any decisions yet,' I blurted out. 'Let's see how things progress.'

As I left the room, I could already sense the eyes following me, busily envisioning the wedding sherwani (suit).

Wedding Bells

Indeed, Nida proved to be a mature woman. She wore a

perpetual smile, exuded serenity, and possessed a twinkle in her eyes. At forty, she wasn't just any woman seeking marriage; she displayed genuine aspirations. Her admiration for my journey, deeming it 'inspiring', felt truly sincere.

To deepen our understanding of each other, I proposed a few additional video calls. 'If you're comfortable with it,' I hastily added, 'and, of course, if your parents approve.'

And so, one of the most remarkable journeys of my life began. The calls persisted for three months, back and forth. Finally, in March, Nida embarked on the journey from Dubai to meet me in person for the first time.

In that moment, I knew I had made the finest decision of my life. We mutually agreed to promptly proceed with our engagement. On 2 April 2021, Ammi's cherished dream became a reality.

* * *

My perspective on Ammi's persistent marriage proposals transformed. Instead of annoyance, I now felt nothing but gratitude. Without her unwavering push, I would have never even considered the idea of marriage.

From that point onward, the next few months unfolded like a fairytale. Following our engagement, Nida returned to Dubai to bid farewell to her job. However, our newfound joy kept us constantly connected, with distance only making our hearts grow fonder. We joyfully occupied our time with the delightful complexities of choosing outfits for the *walima* (post-wedding celebration).

Finally, after two months of virtual courtship, the time came for Nida to permanently return to Mumbai, just three weeks before our wedding day. According to Islamic customs, the bride and groom are not allowed to meet for at least a month before the wedding. However, we found ourselves meeting almost every single day. We happily immersed ourselves in wedding preparations—selecting outfits, jewellery and gifts for both families. The lists seemed endless but working on them was incredibly enjoyable. From choosing each dress to buying wedding rings for one another, we did everything as a couple. It was astonishing how aligned our choices were, whether it was shopping or food preferences.

Compiling the guest list proved challenging. With Covid-19 still a reality and gathering restrictions in place, along with the heavy monsoon rains and flooding in Mumbai, the weather added to our concerns.

On 30 July 2021, our wedding day arrived, a date for which I will forever thank God! It was the day I was blessed with a wonderful and kind-hearted wife. Our nikah (marriage vows) ceremony took place on that bright and clear day, arranged after the evening prayers. I will never forget the moment when I saw the Qazi (priest) entering the wedding venue. It felt like a scene straight out of the Bollywood movies I had watched as a boy. The Qazi recited verses from the Holy Quran, and we, the bride and groom, accepted the vows by saying the two magical words, '*qubool hai*', aloud three times. The Qazi first took the vows from my beautiful bride and then from me.

This was a dream I hadn't even dared to dream, and yet here it was, unfolding right before my eyes. As Nida entered the wedding venue as my wife, I couldn't help but feel immensely proud and deeply satisfied to have this amazing partner in my life.

On 31 July 2021, the day after our nikah, we celebrated our walima. Traditionally, the wedding banquet is organised by the groom's family to commemorate the union. For us, the best part of this incredible day was that Nida and I personally handled every single arrangement—the menu, decorations, wardrobe and guest list. It was a labour of love that we were witnessing coming to fruition. And by the grace of God, there was no rain!

As each guest arrived at the event, I felt overwhelmed with gratitude. Nida warmly greeted and welcomed every guest, genuinely happy and proud to meet the people I knew. She couldn't stop expressing her gratitude to Dr Bhave!

As the evening progressed, it was heartening to witness the abundance of love and joy surrounding us. 'We have done this beautifully,' I whispered to a radiant Nida. While enjoying a grand dinner with our close family, their blessings for a happily married life resonated deeply within me.

Soon, Nida started joining me on my daily runs. Initially, she would walk-jog. On 15 August 2021, we ran our first 10K together: the 10-kilometre at Powai Hiranandani. It was a memorable first.

Indeed, it was only after getting married that I realised the importance of many firsts—the first Eid, first Diwali, and birthdays all took on a new significance. The year 2021 had been entirely different and exceptionally special. It was a year that taught me how much richer life can be with a great companion by your side.

Training Seriously Again

In 2022, Comrades once again consumed my thoughts as I began training rigorously. Soon after, I participated in the Delhi full marathon, the Aegis Federal Life Insurance New Delhi Marathon, which also served as the national try-outs. I achieved an impressive time of 3.37 minutes, securing a commendable rank in my age group.

With the marathon behind me, my entire focus shifted to Comrades. I eagerly desired to take Nida to South Africa to witness one of the world's most highly anticipated ultra-races.

Meanwhile, Virtus had plans to establish a standalone performance centre. Determinedly, I worked on developing a business plan with a franchise model. After careful consideration, we chose a location in Andheri, Mumbai, and commenced the fit-out process.

Our goal was clear—to create a specialised fitness centre catering to individuals recovering from serious illnesses like cancer, focusing on fitness for the specially abled and senior citizens. It would be a haven where people could feel comfortable and at ease, free from any apprehension or intimidation that often accompanies athletic environments. Our dedicated trainers would possess an understanding of each individual's unique needs, crafting personalised programmes tailored to suit their requirements. It was a cherished dream and one close to my heart.

But life had other plans. Just when I believed I had complete control over my life, reality reminded me that I had been living under an illusion.

24

CANCER, AGAIN

In May, amidst an incredibly busy first half of the year, a small blister appeared on the left side of my cheek. The consumption of spicy food intensified the burning sensation. Despite being prescribed antibiotics, none of the treatments seemed to alleviate the issue. Eventually, I sought the expertise of an oral specialist at Mumbai's Kokilaben Dhirubhai Ambani Hospital. Following a punch biopsy, an unsettling truth was revealed—the blister was malignant.

Once again, I found myself confronting a familiar foe. Despite eight years of being free from cancer, I was now embarking on another arduous battle. It was a distinction to bear, a person who had experienced the development of two distinct cancers within a single lifetime. Even the doctors, particularly Dr Abhay Bhave and Dr Shashikant Apte, who had treated my leukaemia, were astounded. If I could possess two different blood groups in one lifetime, why not two different cancers?

This time, the diagnosis was Squamous Cell Carcinoma of the left buccal mucosa.

Thus, the relentless pursuit of the finest doctor and the most effective treatment commenced anew. Fortunately, the esteemed oncologist Dr Sultan Pradhan agreed to take charge of my case.

* * *

2 June 2022. I underwent facial surgery, during which two of my lymph nodes tested positive. Fighting leukaemia for the last fifteen years was a solo battle. But this time, immediately post my surgery, it was different. The hospital room was flooded with people—Nida, my mother-in-law, my two aunts, Nida's sisters and my brothers-in-law and several kids. I feel truly blessed to have such a huge family to support me through my treatment.

The difficult times seemed to ease up. I felt my strength build; I felt pepped up to fight this battle. Despite this setback, my fitness levels facilitated a swift recovery, allowing me to be discharged within a week. The surgical wounds took three weeks to heal. Under the guidance of Dr Vinay Babu at Mumbai's P.D. Hinduja Hospital, we commenced low-dose concurrent chemotherapy and radiation treatment.

The chemotherapy entailed six cycles, synchronised with radiation therapy, necessitating weekly admissions to a daycare facility.

The radiation treatment was scheduled for a total of 33 cycles over seven weeks. Remarkably, each session lasted a mere 10 to 15 minutes as the process was relatively painless and effortless.

This cancer diagnosis arrived just ten months into our marriage. Nida and I were resolute in maximising the time we had together. Like any couple, we yearned for a carefree existence, unburdened by the looming disease.

Yet, we remained acutely aware of the fleeting nature of time. We were consumed by a desire to forge enduring memories. Rather than waiting for the perfect moment, we seized every opportunity that presented itself amidst the treatments. Following the radiation sessions, we ventured out to nearby cafes, relishing shared laughter over steaming cups of coffee. Occasionally, we indulged in shopping for sports attire and equipment. Together, we actively crafted memories, treasuring the invaluable time in each other's company.

Believing that the worst was behind us, we were oblivious to the trials that still lay ahead.

* * *

'I'm well acquainted with radiation,' I confidently assured Nida, 'I've undergone ten radiations on my skull and ten radiations in my testis. I didn't experience any major side effects.'

However, this time, things took an unexpected turn.

Given the combination of chemotherapy and radiation, I had been forewarned about the potential for severe side effects, including mouth blisters, sores and overall oral infections. But no amount of caution could have prepared me for what lay ahead.

Two weeks after commencing the radiation sessions, my entire mouth became covered in blisters. Even the act of sipping water caused excruciating pain. Although I was prescribed antiseptic and anti-inflammatory gargles, the anguish persisted as my mouth could barely open beyond two centimetres.

In most cases like mine, a nasal tube or direct stomach incision would be necessary for nutrition through tube feeding.

'I won't permit any more tubes to be inserted,' I made a resolution to myself.

I attempted to sip orange juice but screamed as my mouth felt ablaze.

Fresh fruit juices were out of the question. Citrus juices were even worse.

Khichdi (lentil and rice porridge), milk, custard, extra-soft bread pudding and jelly were tolerable. Dal (lentil) soups and milk *sevaiyya* (sweet milk and rice porridge) were highly preferred.

'You used to make my favourite dessert only on Eid,' I remarked to Nida and Ammi in jest. 'Now, I can relish it as often as I desire.'

Yet, my menu was limited.

Nevertheless, I persisted.

The situation only worsened – severe tightness in the mouth accompanied by intense discomfort on the left side of my neck. Sleepless nights that felt interminable. Painful days that stretched on. Each day revolved around the sole objective of consuming some liquid, as my saliva production had ceased and my mouth felt parched as bone.

Yet, I remained resolute.

'No matter what, I won't allow them to insert a tube,' I reassured myself steadfastly, 'I will continue to eat through my mouth.'

Finally, the entire treatment concluded. Allah has been merciful. I managed to endure.

This time, I believed that God had doubled my blessings. I wasn't alone. Nida stood by my side. I constantly uttered this prayer, 'Allah, I cannot express enough gratitude for sending Nida into my life.'

This lady warrior remained by my side from the moment of diagnosis, through surgeries, and every single radiation session. When I battled leukaemia, I fought alone. But this time, I had a companion and an unwavering wellspring of moral support. I had my best friend. And it made an immeasurable difference. Regardless of how bleak the circumstances appeared, I perpetually felt blessed to have Nida beside me.

Well Again. Almost!

20 August 2022. A sunny Saturday morning greeted us. It marked the final radiation session. The chemotherapy had long been completed. I made a special request to have a photograph taken with the entire radiology team. Dr Vinay Babu kindly acquiesced and even permitted us to pose with Hinduja's state-of-the-art radiology technology.

Dr Babu had not only been remarkably kind but also exhibited exceptional patience and skill. Despite the bustling crowd and chaotic atmosphere, his team's coordination remained flawlessly synchronised. Dr Babu took the initiative to ensure that every patient, including myself, had a weekly physical examination, in my case, an oral examination.

On that last day, Dr Babu informed me of a minor mouth infection. He prescribed an antibiotic and advised me to schedule appointments once every two weeks.

'It will take three to six months for the side effects of radiation to completely diminish,' he explained.

Dr Pradhan was also notified of the completion of my treatment. His office responded that we would only need to return for a scan after 90 days. That meant I was free until November, to be precise, its second week.

Our hearts brimmed with joy!

* * *

I had suffered a significant loss of muscle mass, leaving my body at its weakest state in over a decade. Nevertheless, my spirit remained content. I chose to stay home for a couple of weeks and gradually initiate gentle treadmill walks.

By mid-September, both Nida and I were yearning for some fresh air.

'Let's resume walking outdoors,' I proposed.

We opted for Ismail Yusuf College in Jogeshwari East, Mumbai, just a short distance from our home. The campus was nestled amidst hills and dense forests, and would remain undisturbed in the evenings. Additionally, it boasted a well-maintained tar road, devoid of potholes, making our walks effortless. The air resonated with the cheerful chirping of birds, while squirrels darted around.

I felt revitalised.

Initially, our target was to walk at a pace of four kilometres per hour. Gradually, both Nida and I managed to alternate between jogging and walking, covering a distance of seven kilometres per hour. I could sense my strength returning.

Our evening walks amidst the greenery became our sanctuary. We replenished ourselves by sipping fresh tender coconut water just outside the campus. On our way back, we strolled along the bustling station road, immersing ourselves in the vibrant market activity. Nida and I became a regular husband-and-wife duo, purchasing fruits, vegetables, or flowers.

Marriage had a positive impact on me.

Even Sunday morning trips to the supermarket became a cherished household ritual. First, we gathered the necessary household items and then visited the speciality store for organic groceries. And, of course, we never missed the opportunity to enjoy a cup of coffee. We concluded our outing with a leisurely walk at Hiranandani Powai, as Sundays were typically pleasant and breezy.

'I had a delightful Sunday morning,' became my customary remark during the drive back home.

Marriage truly benefited me.

Those three months passed like a gentle breeze.

* * *

Timed perfectly for Dr Pradhan's scheduled scan, by the second week of November, my ear began to ache and opening my jaw became increasingly difficult. We swiftly repeated the scan.

The report delivered alarming news—the cancer had spread from the back of my jaw to the lungs and spine.

Dr Pradhan prescribed chemotherapy alongside oral medication. However, desiring additional opinions and alternative treatment options, we sought advice elsewhere.

I consulted Dr Bhave once more, and the name of a respected medical oncologist, Dr Nilesh Lokeshwar, repeatedly emerged. We scheduled an appointment at Mumbai's Lilavati Hospital and Research Centre. In the meantime, the other doctors advised starting a combination of immunotherapy and chemotherapy.

Dr Lokeshwar requested a test to determine the effectiveness of immunotherapy due to its cost. The test results proved positive, and Dr Lokeshwar recommended commencing with immunotherapy alone, forgoing chemotherapy. He believed there was a good chance that immunotherapy would be effective. The plan involved three cycles of immunotherapy, followed by a repeat scan.

A week after the initial cycle, I developed rashes. The dermatologist prescribed an antihistamine, which resolved the issue.

The second cycle took place after 21 days. I experienced a fever, severe dysentery, and nausea. Pinpointing the exact cause proved challenging, just as finding relief did. I rapidly lost five kilogrammes, unable to retain anything beyond a small amount of liquids.

Finally, I completed the third cycle.

Dr Lokeshwar conducted another scan.

Once again, the report delivered unwelcome news—the cancer was spreading. Chemotherapy appeared to be the sole option. Without hesitation, I promptly admitted myself to Lilavati Hospital.

25

TURN TO THE COWS FOR HELP

8 February 2023. The first cycle of chemotherapy began with a slightly reduced dosage to assess my body's reaction. Concurrently, I endured a severe back spasm. Upon discharge on the third day, I discovered that I could no longer walk. I became dependent on a wheelchair, waiting for the car.

During the journey back, I contemplated our life together and expressed to Nida, 'Transitioning from one chemotherapy to the next, from one cancer to another, we can't continue like this. Perhaps we should explore alternative treatments,' I muttered.

The idea lingered in my mind, and I sought the advice of my old friend, Dr Bhave. He wholeheartedly agreed that it was an opportune time to consider other options.

The following days were consumed by thorough research on alternative cancer treatments. To my surprise, there were numerous choices available in India. Despite living with cancer for many years, I had never delved into this realm before. Bengaluru emerged as a prominent hub, and Shimoga in Karnataka presented potential possibilities.

As if life had its plans waiting for me, I reconnected with an old friend who introduced me to someone I instinctively trusted. He recommended a book called *Holy Cancer* by Amit Vaidya, featuring the inspiring story of a cancer survivor at Shree RMD Ayurved College and Hospital in Vaghaldhara near Valsad, Gujarat.

A chord resonated within me, and I felt an instant connection. Further research affirmed the positive reputation of the facility in Gujarat.

Uncertain of Nida's response, I asked, 'Should we give it a try?'

'I will accompany you,' she replied, 'But first, consult your doctors.'

Without hesitation, I picked up the phone and received approval from my doctors. We contacted RMD, secured our accommodation, and made the commitment. The decision was made.

We patiently waited for 21 days, allowing the chemotherapy drugs to completely leave my system. Then, my body would be ready for something new—a fresh start.

* * *

6 March 2023. RMD proved to be a unique hospital, where stays were required for a minimum of eight to 10 days. The entire treatment was provided free of charge for patients, with just a nominal fee of one rupee per day for the accompanying attendant.

The head doctor checked us in with remarkable honesty, saying, 'The treatment may work for some and not for others. It's simply a matter of belief and giving it a try.'

In my heart, I had yearned to try something different. Nineteen years of radiation and chemotherapy, and yet, relapse after relapse!

'I will give it a try,' I replied.

We embarked on our journey to Gujarat, unsure of what awaited us. With an inflamed tumour in my lumbar region, walking became impossible. Would I be confined to a wheelchair? At that moment, all my doubts seemed to dissipate. The decision to stay was spontaneous. We sent the car back home with the driver and committed ourselves to eight days there.

They explained a nutrition plan to me, which appeared quite restrictive. However, I resolved to give this treatment approach a sincere attempt. I was ready to do whatever was required, without hesitation.

The next morning, my challenge began. The day commenced with Panchagavya, a 50 ml shot to be consumed before sunrise. Panchagavya formed the core of the therapy, consisting of a blend of cow dung, cow urine, milk, curd and wheatgrass powder, all sourced from the indigenous Gir cow. The Gir cow, recognised by its distinctive hump, also provided the native A2 milk renowned worldwide for its numerous benefits. I gulped it down!

Throughout the day, I received several kadhas (herbal liquid nutraceuticals) and Ayurvedic and herbal tablets. The doctor explained, 'The purpose of spending 10 days here is to learn how to make the kadhas and the Panchagavya. You will have to continue taking them for at least a minimum of two years.'

I was instructed to follow a nutritional plan based on Chauvihar, a diet pattern primarily observed by the Jain community. Chauvihar dictated abstaining from food and drink (except water and milk) from sunset until sunrise.

'Isn't it an incredible experience?' I said to Nida as we concluded Day 1. The lifestyle change was as new to her as it was to me.

In the following days, we visited the centre's cowshed, home to approximately 400 Gir cows. The energy in the gaushala (cowshed) was both vibrant and soothing. I reached out to touch the forehead of one of the cows, and she began licking my hand.

'It's a blessing,' the man in charge smiled.

'We will come again before we leave and treat them to some sweet jaggery,' Nida spontaneously replied.

The remaining days were spent learning to embrace the simple yet enriching lifestyle. I acquired knowledge on creating different food colours and the significance and preparation of Panchagavya. I also learned to make the *lep* (ointment or gel) using products derived from cows. Twice a day, I applied it to the areas with tumours and sat in the sun for 20 minutes. The seven days flew by.

On the second last day, I said to Nida, 'Tomorrow we will depart, carrying these beautiful experiences with us.' It immediately reminded us to visit the gaushala and fulfil our promise to the cows.

As we bid farewell on the eighth day, a sense of positivity and gratitude filled both of us.

* * *

13 March 2023. Upon returning to Mumbai, we made a firm commitment to continue with this treatment regimen. We obtained a month's supply of medications, along with fresh groceries and desi cow ghee from RMD.

Now, my initial challenge was to find desi cows in Mumbai. However, it wasn't just milk that I required. I needed a source that could provide fresh milk, cow urine and cow dung every morning before 6 a.m. The first few days were spent in futile searches.

Then, Mr Praful Mungi, a client of Virtus who owned a farmhouse in Nashik with six desi cows reached out to me, hoping he could provide a lead.

'Shiraz, you're most welcome to come and stay here for as long as you need,' the gracious voice on the other end offered.

Nida and I discussed it, and surprisingly, we felt prepared to make the move without hesitation. A profound sense of gratitude engulfed me. I was incredibly fortunate to have such supportive individuals in my life—true angels.

I called Dr Bhave to inform him that I was back in town but might need to relocate once again. Unexpectedly, Dr Bhave mentioned that one of his patients had a cowshed in Goregaon, Mumbai, which was conveniently close to my place.

My friend Nitin inspected the facility, and the owners were cooperative and willing to meet my daily requirements for desi cow products.

Thanks to this sudden turn of events, the need to relocate to Nasik was no longer necessary. Help appeared out of nowhere.

'I am truly blessed,' I whispered to myself. 'Thank you, God.'

26

THE FIGHT CONTINUES, BUT I WILL WIN

I was determined to continue this strict regime with all its concoctions, but as usual, life had other plans. The pain in my spine shot up so much that I was unable to move from my bed.

I was rushed to Hinduja Hospital where Dr Babu recommended a pelvic MRI urgently followed by five rounds of localised radiation to reduce pain. Back home, the flaring pain made the strict Ayurveda regimen almost impossible to follow. I needed urgent help—the disease was spreading fast. Ayurveda had to wait.

The doctors recommended targeted therapy. I agreed because I wanted to get my mobility back on track first. It was my utmost priority.

Nida and I met with Dr Sevanti Limaye at Sir H.N. Reliance Foundation Hospital and were impressed with her well-defined protocol which began with a genetic analysis. 'Do a cancer track analysis every month. This will avoid the PET scan and give us a clear direction,' she advised.

We started with targeted therapy combined with chemotherapy for six weeks. After a year of disappointing

PET scan reports, finally, for the first time, the scan showed that the tumour has shrunk. 'It's working,' a relieved Nida said to me with a smile. 'It will take another year perhaps but, we will go on. I feel a change,' I smiled back. We both came out feeling positive.

* * *

We feel equally invested in this fight. It's been over a year since the diagnosis in May 2022. When you start an ultra-distance race like the Comrades, you don't know what the hurdles will be. But your mind is prepared to take up any challenge—be it the steep uphill climb and the aggressive downhill walk, or to just keep one foot in front of the other and remain strong and focused. I am running my 'personal' Comrades with this ailment. Right now, it's a steep uphill climb for me, a slow one. I continue to put one foot in front of the other—one chemotherapy after another. I remain strong, stay focused and believe in Allah. I will finally see the finish line.

I will come out victorious, beating cancer once again.

* * *

Each one of us has calculated lives to live. Our laughter, our tears and even our breaths are calculated with arithmetic precision. But still, we just live on.

We meander through our days grumbling and complaining about the trivial. We wake up each morning without being grateful for having been blessed with yet another sunrise, yet another opportunity to do the very best we can. We stumble on unaware of life's plans.

Life certainly has its plans. For each one of us.

My life has taught me immensely. When life offers smiles and sunshine, let happiness flood through you. Be humble and be kind enough to spread the joy. All it takes is a kind word here and a small action there. Whenever I have felt blessed, I have always shared my blessings. And the universe has blessed me abundantly in return.

Life has taught me that before you blink, the course ahead will change. It will turn around and take you to the darkest spots. But it will be your acts of kindness, the people whose lives you've touched that will come to your rescue. They are the people who will be your guardian angels. They will protect you. They will be there for you in your darkest moments.

I may have spent half my life battling cancer. But I have also spent my life living each moment—celebrating my mind, body and spirit through my fitness and celebrating success through Virtus. Throughout the journey, I have discovered guardian angels that have appeared as if by magic—clients who have helped financially, friends who have become family and even my new family that stands by me each day.

This fight against cancer is not done yet. I have yet to run the ultimate human race, the Comrades. Run it, I must. I must cross the finish line. The Comrades will be my ultimate HUMANE race. I seek your blessings.

27

UNTIL WE MEET AGAIN, SHIRAZ

Shiraz's battle with cancer began at Lilavati Hospital in 2004 when it was diagnosed by Dr Bhave that he was suffering from Acute Lymphoblastic Leukaemia (A.L.L.). Tragically, it concluded there too in September 2023, with Dr Bhave, now a close friend, delivering the devastating prognosis of his limited time remaining.

This last chapter, which Shiraz ideally should have written, has fallen on my lap to complete, and I am writing it after his passing. As his wife and closest confidante, I witnessed his last days till his last breath. It was an earth-shattering experience for me, but I could handle it purely because of the courage and energy that Shiraz inspired in me.

Here's an account of how it all panned out in the end.

It was May 2023 and Shiraz was under the treatment of Dr Sewanti Limaye from Sir H.N Reliance Foundation Hospital. At that time, we had no inkling that matters would only get worse.

Post a PET scan, biopsy and various other tests, Shiraz was prescribed chemotherapy and targeted therapy combinations. However, unlike immunotherapy, which was given every 21 days, this therapy was given every week. And hence the first six cycles were completed in one-and-a-half months. Shiraz was due for the next PET scan in June to check the effect of the therapies administered. Since Shiraz was confined to bed since March 2023, I used to take him for weekly treatment by ambulance.

And finally, the day that we were waiting for more than a year had arrived. Much to our relief, Shiraz's health showed marginal improvement with the report revealing the shrinking of some of the tumours. When we met Dr Limaye, she informed us that though the treatment needed to be prolonged, Shiraz was responding to the treatment.

Shiraz and I were on cloud nine. We finally saw a ray of hope and started to plan our life. We were confident that the sad days were about to get over and we would be able to live our lives like any other couple. That was one of the happiest moments in my life. We decided to remain positive and patient with the treatment and continue for as long as required. We contacted everyone close to us, who were equally concerned and were praying hard for Shiraz's health, to inform them about the report and thanked everyone for keeping Shiraz in their prayers.

Shiraz was doing good, eating well and above all, was happy. He said, 'I have a feeling that I will be able to sit at least in the co-driver's seat and go for drives with you, Nida, and enjoy our coffee together once again.' We started making plans, deciding that once Shiraz got better, the first place we would go together would be to perform Umrah.

* * *

Twist in the tale

Things were good. However, there came a twist in the story yet again. Since July 2023, Shiraz started experiencing continuous shooting pain in his lower back even when immobile. It got more intense as days went by, spreading to his thighs. It reached a point when Shiraz could not even fold his legs without the help of both his hands. We knew that an MRI done earlier had revealed that Shiraz had burst fractures in his spine. This term was completely new, at least to me, and the doctor had explained that a few of Shiraz's vertebrae had burst due to the growth of the tumours in his spine.

Despite the nagging pain in his lower back, Shiraz and I were still thinking positively, conjecturing that maybe the pain had increased due to the shrinking of the tumours and the fracture. The doctor increased the dosage of his painkillers; some were even administered intravenously during our weekly visits for therapies. However, there was no relief from the pain.

Yet, Shiraz embodied the spirit of resilience. Throughout this harrowing journey, what struck me most was his unwavering determination to embrace life, despite enduring unimaginable pain. Not once did I hear him utter a word of resignation or express a desire to surrender to the ordeal.

This steadfast resolve was truly remarkable, especially considering Shiraz's tumultuous medical history. Despite being declared fully cured following a gruelling bone marrow transplant, a mere nine months into our marriage, a new form of cancer surfaced. Astonishingly, this wasn't a relapse; rather, it was an entirely distinct manifestation. Even the doctors were astounded by Shiraz's case, witnessing a rare occurrence where an individual grappled with two distinct types of cancer within a single lifetime.

Despite Shiraz's enduring pain and numerous medications, we cherished each moment together with immense joy. Even as his condition worsened, we continued to savour our outings, shopping trips, coffee dates, and walks/runs at Ismail Yusuf College until December 2022.

Throughout July and August 2023, Shiraz endured relentless agony. Despite alterations in treatment to mitigate his suffering, relief remained elusive. Consequently, another PET scan and Cancer Track Analysis became imperative. Swiftly, I arranged a blood test and PET scan, and eagerly awaited the results.

At the end of August 2023, we arranged a blood test for Cancer Track Analysis. As September first, Shiraz's birthday month, dawned, I anticipated joy, unaware of the challenges ahead. Despite Shiraz's agony, we made it to the hospital for the PET scan. Witnessing his pain, I stayed by his side during the scan, disregarding the doctors' requests to leave. After the ordeal, we returned home, eagerly awaiting the report. Though I promptly scheduled doctor appointments for the following day, we could only secure one for the day after.

On September 3, I met with Dr Limaye to review the report. Her initial words, 'The disease has increased,' left me stunned and unsure how to respond. As she meticulously examined the report, a heavy silence enveloped the room. Dr Limaye conveyed that the disease had advanced, still affecting Shiraz's spine and lungs. Exploring all options, she recommended oral chemotherapy. She prescribed several tablets, some to be taken weekly.

That day marked the first time I harboured doubts about Shiraz's treatment. Uncertainty clouded my thoughts, perhaps due to the altered treatment plan. When I informed Shiraz about it, his simple plea, 'Please come back home,' resonated deeply within me. Feeling adrift, my sole desire was to return home quickly. Upon arrival, Shiraz and I didn't converse much. We shared a meal before I busied myself with household chores while he watched TV, though his focus seemed distant. I administered his medicines and attended to all the tasks as usual, wondering if his calm demeanour masked any underlying concerns.

Later he made me sit and asked me to narrate everything the doctor had told me. He said that as per his experience with cancer, the medicines prescribed may not be helpful for the aggressive type of disease he has. He insisted on speaking with the doctor himself to understand the side effects of the medicines prescribed and if these would show any positive results. I called the doctor even though it was past ten at night as I was desperate to understand what was happening or what was to happen going forward. The doctor answered the call and spoke with Shiraz, advising him that the medicines had worked in certain cases. Hence, we decided to take one tablet at a time to understand the side effects, if any. As per the protocol, Shiraz had to get a blood test done five days after taking the oral chemo to ensure the blood counts were stable.

A few days later, Shiraz expressed a desire to consult a spine specialist in the hope of finding a solution for his discomfort, so as to enable him to sit comfortably in a wheelchair. He confided in me, saying, 'Nida, I'm uncertain about the future, but right now, all I want is to experience the outdoors with you—even if it means being in a wheelchair. I want to create lasting memories together.' I wholeheartedly embraced his wish.

After a referral, we located a spine specialist at Hinduja Hospital. Due to the need for a physical examination, Shiraz's admission became necessary as video consultation wasn't feasible. Upon admission, a battery of tests including X-rays, scans, and blood tests preceded the spine MRI scheduled for the next day. Shiraz, already fatigued, underwent these procedures. We also consulted with Dr Babu, who expressed concern about Shiraz's condition. Despite excruciating pain, Shiraz consented to the spine MRI, though he struggled to rest that night, both from the pain and the anticipation of the test results.

Around 1.30 a.m., just hours before the scheduled MRI, I made the difficult decision to cancel it. Concerned about the potential post-anesthesia pain, I feared Shiraz's discomfort once the effects wore off. Shiraz, too, expressed relief, sharing my apprehensions. We opted to be discharged from the hospital without undergoing the MRI. Upon returning home, I received Shiraz's blood test results, indicating an urgent need for a blood transfusion. Despite our recent hospital visit, Shiraz postponed the procedure for two days due to exhaustion. Given the flexibility of the transfusion location, Shiraz chose Lilavati Hospital for his admission.

On 14 September, I admitted Shiraz to Lilavati Hospital for a blood transfusion under the care of Dr Bhave. After a thorough examination and review of recent reports, Dr Bhave delivered devastating news: 'Shiraz does not have much time.' He advised me to keep Shiraz at home, surrounded by loved ones, as much as possible.

* * *

My Darkest Days Began

The news marked the beginning of my darkest and most sorrowful days. While Shiraz and I were informed to prepare ourselves for what lay ahead, we never anticipated it would come so swiftly. Shiraz was discharged from Lilavati Hospital on September 15. I was advised to consult a nearby general practitioner to discuss Shiraz's medical history in case of an emergency.

It was Shiraz's birthday the next day, September 16. It sure felt like it could be his last birthday with me. After we got back home from the hospital, I requested Shiraz to allow me to invite his team from Virtus to celebrate his birthday. Shiraz asked me to call them home the following week as he wanted to celebrate the day with me. However, I insisted, and Shiraz agreed to invite his Virtus team over. As soon as the clock struck midnight, I could not stop my tears as I wished him.

Shiraz's birthday unfolded in a way none of us could have anticipated. As the Virtus team arrived at our home with cake and snacks to celebrate, they were unprepared for the news Shiraz was about to share. Without hesitation, Shiraz informed them that the doctor had advised him to prepare for the end of life. The team was stunned into silence. Shiraz emphasised the importance of cherishing life and family, expressing his contentment with his journey.

Despite the disappointment of not being able to participate in the Comrades event, he took pride in achieving his goals, inspiring others, and most importantly, facing cancer bravely. Grateful for the remarkable people he had met, he lamented only about the short time he had with me. Expressing his love for me, he said, 'After waiting for so long, I finally found true love in my life. I wanted to reciprocate the love she gave me tenfold, but life has other plans. I will truly miss her.'

The team was not ready to leave and were with us till late evening. I insisted that Shiraz cut the cake the team had brought with them. While Shiraz was cutting the cake, he sang, 'This is my last birthday' to the tune of '*Happy Birthday to me*'. Everyone in the room was in tears.

In the quiet of the night, with only five minutes remaining until the next day, I bid Shiraz a final happy birthday and expressed gratitude for being the most cherished part of my life—the best husband, and above all, my dearest friend.

Though my family was scheduled to join us at our home on Shiraz's birthday, they had to defer it to the next day. Shiraz appeared unwell upon waking, and was having trouble in breathing and speaking. Despite his condition, he greeted the guests briefly. After feeding him breakfast, I joined my family in the living area. Shortly after, my sister emerged to inform me of Shiraz's worsening condition—he had developed a sudden high-grade fever that medication failed to alleviate. Concerned, I waited for signs of improvement, but seeing none after two hours, I hurriedly rushed him to Lilavati Hospital for immediate medical attention the next day after his birthday.

Shiraz was admitted to Lilavati on September 17. His temperature was constantly fluctuating, and he was finding it extremely difficult to breathe. The doctors at Lilavati gave every possible medicine, orally and intravenously to make Shiraz comfortable, but nothing seemed to be working. I had realised by then that this time I would be returning home without Shiraz. All I did during the whole duration of this hospital stay was hold Shiraz's hand and rest my head on his lap. We kept looking at each other as much as possible, keeping in mind that the moment would never return. We had all his clients visiting him to see him for the last time and all of them had tears in their eyes. They could not believe that a person as strong as Shiraz was in this miserable state. But Shiraz greeted everyone and even managed to smile at them. Finally, he passed away peacefully in the wee hours of September 20. I will never forget that moment of watching him take his last breath.

After enduring sixteen months of relentless efforts to save my beloved husband, our journey had come to an end. I'll forever hold onto his last words to me: 'Nida, though my life is fading, my love for you will never diminish. You, and only you, will always be my true love.'

Though Shiraz and I shared just two years with each other, they were undoubtedly the most joyful of my life. He showered me with unconditional love, unwavering support, and boundless encouragement to pursue my dreams. While our time together feels fleeting, especially in these sorrowful days, I am profoundly grateful for the blessing of having Shiraz as my husband. Despite the heartbreak, I find solace in knowing that Shiraz now resides in a world free from tears, pain, and death.

Shiraz harboured a singular ambition: to conquer the formidable Comrades marathon. Regrettably, that dream eluded him. Yet, reflecting on his journey, one realizes his life was a marathon of its own, traversing paths as arduous as any Comrades race. Emerging from the impoverished alleys of Mumbai, he carved out a distinct identity, defying adversity at every turn. Battling cancer relentlessly over two decades, enduring countless treatments and immeasurable discomfort, he not only survived but thrived, establishing a successful company and even taking on marathons post-treatment. Shiraz ran a personal Comrades race unlike any other, embodying resilience, positivity, and unwavering courage.

His indomitable spirit, marked by an infectious smile and steadfast perseverance, remains a beacon of inspiration. Though his physical presence has departed, his spirit endures, stirring the souls of countless admirers. Shiraz exemplified a rare breed, one whose purpose transcends mere existence, imparting invaluable life lessons that linger long after their departure. In my journey alongside him, as both spouse and confidant, I've gleaned profound wisdom, recognising the profound impact of souls like Shiraz on the fabric of existence.

Though I miss him terribly, he will always be my inspiration and protect me wherever he is. Above all, he will always remain my best friend.

Until we meet again, Shiraz!

PART IV

My Angels

FAMILY, AND CLOSE FRIEND

'She meant everything to me'

Kulsum Abdul Wahab Siddiqui
My Ammi

My mother has always been like a friend to me. She always encouraged my interest in sports and told me that I should complete my studies until graduation, regardless of the grades I achieved. She never pressured me or stopped me from participating in sports. She always supported me and meant everything to me.

It was truly heartbreaking to see her sell her jewellery to support our studies. I was particularly saddened when she had to sell her wedding ring to cover my father's medical expenses when he was seriously ill. Unfortunately, he couldn't recover. During that moment, I made a promise to myself and told my mom that I would ensure she got back all the jewellery she had to sell, not just in gold, but also in diamonds.

I eagerly awaited finding a good job, and when I got a job at Marriott, my priority was to fulfil that promise. Every year, at least two times – once on her birthday and once during Diwali, I would take her to her favourite place, Tribhoovandas Bhimji Zaveri at Zaveri Bazaar. I was thrilled that within a few years, I was able to fulfil my promise. I not only bought her gold jewellery but also, diamonds and she wore them proudly for the first time in her life. Seeing her smiling face meant everything to me. I was the happiest son.

However, my mother also wanted me to get married, and due to her persistent persuasion, I eventually found a girl named Nida whom I married. Nida became more of a friend to me than just a wife, and I owe thanks to my mother for pushing me to marry. Six months after our marriage, my mother's health started deteriorating. At that time, she was around 79 years old and had diabetes, arthritis, and related complications.

We had to admit her to Lilavati Hospital in December 2021. I distinctly remember that she was discharged on 31 December, but her health continued to decline. In May, her blood sugar level became dangerously high, leading to a five-day stay in the ICU. After being discharged, she was bedridden and unable to walk. She spent the next four months in excruciating pain in bed.

On 14 September 2022, at 6.05 in the evening, she passed away peacefully while I sat beside her, holding her hand. I was deeply saddened, but at the same time, relieved that she was no longer suffering and had found peace. I will never forget her as a son, and I consider myself not just lucky, but truly blessed to have spent my entire life with her, from the day I was born until the day she passed away. I was fortunate to be there for her when she needed me the most. I was lucky to have the opportunity to fulfil her dreams, just as she had fulfilled mine.

She had very few friends, and one of her closest childhood friends had passed away long ago, so she often felt lonely. However, I was grateful that I was always there for her, taking care of her and making her dreams come true. She was the first person in our family to travel abroad. She had always wanted to visit Dubai and experience travelling by air. I would be very happy to see her smile. What was more important was that I was able to make her smile. My mother was able to see me get married, something, I believe, she had been eagerly waiting for.

'He is such a fighter'

Nida Siddiqui

My Soulmate

When I came in contact with Shiraz, the first thing that struck me was his honesty. He was completely upfront about his history, both medical and personal, and was proud to be known as someone who beat cancer. The fact that he wanted to share his experience and influence others like him showed a very positive aspect of him.

As I got to know him better, we both discovered similarities between us which we never expected to find in another person. And that made our decision to spend our lives together much easier. We had a lovely, intimate wedding with the blessings of both our families.

Everything seemed to be smooth sailing. We were happy in our small family. Shiraz was always supportive and appreciative. Being the businessman that he was, he constantly encouraged me to do my own thing and to have an aim in life.

Last year, cancer raised its head again. I was completely devastated and did not know how to deal with the situation. I was having all kinds of negative thoughts. But Shiraz amazed me once again with his willpower and positive attitude. He was a fighter and I have decided to be one as well. I hope and pray that I continue to face the world with the courage that he showed all his life.

'He will surely emerge victorious!'

Firoz Siddiqui

My Brother

I was the eldest child in our family, and as I grew up, I often witnessed my father engrossed in work while my mother focused solely on household matters. As a result, I used to immerse myself in unstructured play, yearning for a companion with whom I could share toys and spend endless hours playing.

Finally, after a seven-year gap, Shiraz came into our family as my younger brother. At the time of his birth, he was weak. Little did I know that he would transform into a resilient and determined individual, accomplishing everything he set his mind on. Shiraz was ambitious and insistent on following an unmatched work ethic. Despite the challenges we faced as a working-class family, we also created cherished memories together, fostering a deep bond between us.

The true test of courage and patience arrived when Shiraz was initially diagnosed with Acute Lymphoblastic Leukaemia (A.L.L.). From controlling our emotions to making the necessary arrangements to combat this dreadful disease, we faced a daunting journey.

I am grateful that I could assist him during his bone marrow transplant, and I am overjoyed to see how happily married he was in life, albeit for a short period of time. Although Shiraz battled the illness for the longest time, I was confident that he would eventually emerge victorious. But Allah had other plans. He took Shiraz away from us in September 2023.

'Triumph over adversity'

Nitin Rane

Director – Operations, Virtus Wellness Pvt. Ltd

I joined JW Marriott in 2005 as a pool operator, and during that time, Shiraz was my team leader. Through my colleagues, I learned about his diagnosis and was amazed at his enduring energy and zest for life. Shiraz embodied true leadership, constantly inspiring and motivating his team while establishing clear roles, responsibilities and expectations. He had a remarkable ability to uplift those around him. Furthermore, he harboured a long-standing desire to establish his own wellness company and dedicated every ounce of effort to navigating the intricate details of starting a business.

In 2009, Shiraz received news that his cancer had relapsed. Despite this setback, it did not deter him from forging ahead with his entrepreneurial dream, prompting him to resign from his job. He graciously offered me the opportunity to join his business as a site supervisor, a role I happily accepted. Additionally, I took on the responsibility of recruiting exceptional trainers for Virtus. Nilesh was the first personal trainer we hired, marking the inception of Virtus Wellness Private Limited.

From our humble beginnings with just three members, our team has now grown to comprise 40 individuals, training esteemed CEOs and developers within the town. Together, we have completed numerous national and international marathons. Among my most cherished memories with Shiraz is witnessing his relentless spirit as he cycled non-stop for 100 kilometres on his birthday, following a bone marrow transplant. Remarkably, he prepared for this feat in just fourteen weeks!

I have stood by Shiraz through every triumph and tribulation, offering support during his battles with cancer relapses and his subsequent bone marrow transplant. Throughout these arduous journeys, Shiraz consistently demonstrated immense strength, patience and unwavering positivity. My heartfelt prayers go out to his loved ones, now that he is no longer with us. His will was strong till the very end, but God clearly had other plans for him.

DOCTORS

Shiraz – my patient, my trainer, my friend!

Dr Abhay A. Bhave

Hematologist, Lilavati Hospital and Research Centre, Mumbai

There will always be people you meet who deeply impact your life, making you think differently. They make you realise that recovery encompasses more than just medicine and science. Faith, belief, physical fitness and positive thinking are fantastic additions that aid in healing. This is something I observed in the young man I had a long association with, both during his illness and when he was in remission, free from his disease.

In my field of haematology, success and failure are often seen as endpoints. However, with Shiraz Siddiqui, his journey through his disease (or diseases!) was a series of events that taught and enlightened me. He only desired to overcome against all odds, all the while wearing a smile, never blaming the Almighty for his illness.

While people often break down and curse their maker for giving them a disease, Shiraz didn't. He embraced each phase of his illness as a challenge. I must add that his physical fitness and mental fortitude carried him through thick and thin, not just once, but time and time again. Why would God test someone so frequently with disease? Perhaps God knew that certain individuals could handle it better and become role models for others facing similar predicaments. I can only express gratitude for my destiny, allowing me to treat and closely observe a man who defied all odds in his singular desire—t\o triumph. His attitude, fitness, ability to organise funds for his treatment, and quick decision-making skills were all admirable traits.

His medical journey is akin to a long poem, with numerous verses depicting different events and outcomes that culminate in victory time and again. It's like a batsman fearlessly hitting the ball on a treacherous pitch!

This is the story of a young man who appeared fit as he awaited his diagnosis in the outpatient department. However, to my dismay, his physical examination and peripheral blood smear under the microscope raised suspicions of the worst. I was convinced that I was dealing with blood cancer.

While we learn to conceal our emotions over time, it's always challenging to deliver bad news to a good person. No one prepares us for this in our formative years. Even for me, it was difficult to inform this very fit individual about his blood cancer diagnosis, fully expecting him to disbelieve me. After all, we had only just met.

However, the truth had to be told, and to my surprise, instead of a shocking response, I received a small smile (perhaps he had anticipated it after reading his earlier blood report) and a look that conveyed a sense of calmness, as if to say, 'No worries, I will handle it.' He was diagnosed with acute lymphatic leukaemia.

Fortunately, there were no poor predictive markers, making this a disease worth treating. The results of treating this disease in children are better than in adults, but we have witnessed many success stories among adults as well. I hope to impress upon the readers of this book and chapter that Shiraz is one such remarkable success story. He faced the diagnosis courageously and after discussions, he said he needed time to consider the treatment site, finances and the treating doctor. We presented him with various options and I thought I had seen the last of him.

Just a few days later, he was admitted under my care for treatment, and he appeared to be in good spirits, ready to conquer the disease. He had a relatively good prognosis, with the only disadvantage being his age, but he possessed a significant advantage in terms of physical and mental fitness.

We initiated his chemotherapy, which resulted in a lengthy hospital stay. At the end of it all, he achieved remission within a month. He never gave up on his fitness training and maintained a positive attitude even when unwell, prompting me to call him 'the smiling assassin of his disease!'

He underwent chemotherapy for the next two years and six months, experiencing both favourable and challenging events along the way. However, at the culmination of this relentless chemotherapy, he defeated his cancer. He remained disease-free and in complete remission.

He returned to a normal life and work routine, keeping me informed about his blood tests. He aimed to maintain his fitness while helping his clients stay fit and even managed to expand his business. It seemed like he was on track to becoming a great success story.

Unfortunately, approximately four years later, he experienced similar symptoms to when he was first diagnosed, and a repeat blood test raised suspicions of a relapse of his leukaemia. A bone marrow test confirmed it.

This was a significant setback for both of us, as we had become good friends, and he was now my trainer too. (While I am happy to write that he conquered this setback as well, please read until the end when destiny played a different hand.)

As expected, Shiraz wasn't ready to let go, especially now that he had started building an empire with his fitness training. Medically, when leukaemia relapses after two or more years and the genetic markers are not risky, the response to treatment is still favourable. Most patients lose interest and blame their destiny for the relapse, often becoming lost to follow-up. But not our Shiraz!

We decided to restart the treatment regimen, and once again, he conquered the disease, completing his course of chemotherapy over two years. Despite the toll it took on his body, he returned to action with no detectable residual disease in his blood and bone marrow. By this point, I was in awe of this person. What a Superman! Not once, but twice, and without much complaint, he maintained his fitness by exercising even during his chemotherapy sessions!

After the leukaemia was eradicated, we discussed the possibility of a bone marrow transplantation. This procedure allows us to replace the patient's bone marrow with cells from a partially matched donor, resulting in a 'chimaera'—a patient whose characteristics remain the same, but their blood cells originate from the donor. The perceived risk of leukaemia recurrence was high at this point.

But God had more tests in store. Shiraz's only brother was not a perfect match for bone marrow donation, and his mother was not a suitable candidate due to her age and other medical issues. Finding a donor from the registry proved challenging, as there were not many listed at that time (fortunately, we now have a larger pool of donors on the registry). We had to abandon the idea of a transplant and leave it to God and Shiraz's destiny.

Around four years into his second remission (which meant a decade had passed since his initial diagnosis), Shiraz had become a prolific fitness entrepreneur, guide and guru. However, the fear of relapse lingered in the back of our minds. During a casual discussion one evening, that fear became palpable. It had been almost four years since his second treatment—around the same time that the disease had returned the last time. He grew increasingly anxious, evident from the number of phone calls and false alarms regarding symptoms.

We decided to seek the opinion of my dear friend, Dr Shashikant Apte, at Sahyadri Hospital in Pune, regarding the possibility of a half-match transplant from Shiraz's brother. Dr Apte informed us that advancements in science made this feasible. He promptly reassessed Shiraz and his brother for HLA matching and fitness for transplantation. Eventually, he delivered the positive verdict that transplanting Shiraz with cells from his half-matched biological brother was a viable option. Now was the time to entrust Shiraz to the care and management of Dr Apte. Of course, I was just a phone call away. So, for the first time, we proceeded with the curative option of bone marrow transplantation in Pune.

Shiraz underwent the procedure with great determination, even practising Tai Chi on the day of the transplant! He fared exceptionally well, engrafting sooner than expected, and eventually left the transplant room to return to Mumbai for rest and rehabilitation. He remained under the supervision of Dr Apte.

But no, this story doesn't conclude with 'and they all lived happily ever after!' Just when we thought we had won the war, another battle emerged. Shiraz came to me complaining of pain in his mouth. An ulcer had developed, and although we attempted some local applications for relief, it persisted. We consulted an oral surgeon, and to my disbelief, the biopsy from that site revealed an unrelated second primary malignancy—buccal squamous cell carcinoma. How cruel can fate and destiny be to someone? It was a tremendous shock for me but not for Shiraz. He simply said, 'I can, cer (sir)!' (pun intended). He commenced chemotherapy with a medical oncologist.

What a journey, what a man, what a human being!

His temperament, nature, and zeal for fitness made Shiraz a prime example of Charles Darwin's theory—survival of the fittest. I am convinced that his fitness, both mentally and physically, carried him through this incredibly tough period. He not only won awards and led campaigns but, more importantly, captured hearts.

Unfortunately, fate was cruel, and took Shiraz away from us in September 2023. But I must say, long live such icons!

He is truly a superstar!

Dr Kalpana Rao
Corporate and Expat Physician

I want to thank God for introducing such a wonderful human being into my life. Not everyone is as fortunate as I am, but whoever reads this book would be lucky to have known him.

Shiraz and I met at JW Marriott Juhu in 2002. He was working at the gym and fitness centre, while I was the in-house doctor. He amazed me with his extensive knowledge of health and the human body.

In 2004, he came to me with low haemoglobin levels, so I started him on iron injections. However, they did not work. I then referred him to Dr Tushar Shah, a physician, who treated him for fifteen days, but his condition did not improve significantly. We decided to conduct further tests, and that evening, I called Shiraz to deliver the diagnosis of leukaemia.

I can never forget that day. I was shocked when he remained calm on the other end of the phone and said, 'It's okay, it's just another diagnosis, and we will treat it.' Meanwhile, I was emotionally shaken and felt ashamed of myself.

From that moment on, I had no idea that I would look up to Shiraz in awe. His chemotherapy sessions, hospitalisations, testicular cancer a few years later, and bone marrow transplant—throughout it all, we stayed in touch, and he remained full of life and energy.

He changed my perception of life. I prayed to God, expressing my gratitude if I could become at least one per cent of what Shiraz is, mentally, emotionally and physically. All specialists and doctors were now consulting Shiraz for fitness advice.

Later, we shared another workplace at D'Decor, thanks to Shiraz, where we would meet twice a month. He was always encouraging me and everyone else to prioritise fitness (doctors need a BIG push for that!).

I reminisce about those joyful days when Shiraz was cancer-free, participating in marathons, and aspiring to compete in the Iron Man competition. His unwavering focus on running, cycling and swimming was truly inspiring. When he got married, I had the pleasure of meeting him and his wife Nida in Goa. However, I was taken aback when he informed me about his oral cancer diagnosis.

During a video chat with Shiraz, I noticed his high energy and constant smile, radiating positivity even during his chemotherapy and post-surgery. I can't help but wonder if he was truly human! I am convinced that I have encountered a superhero in my life. Shiraz, you were God's chosen one, illuminating our lives. May you always be blessed wherever you are!

VIRTUS CLIENTS

Virtus was established in April 2010 with two revenue streams: corporate wellness programmes and personal training for High-Net-Worth Individuals (HNIs). Throughout my eight-year tenure at JW Marriott, I not only gained valuable experience but also earned the respect of my clients. Trust played a crucial role, as many clients trusted me to guide them towards healthier lives. They had confidence in my expertise. Therefore, upon launching Virtus, I made it a priority to impart this knowledge to all the personal trainers we hired. It was essential for me to ensure that my employees felt they were continuously learning and developing alongside their work. This approach allowed me to focus on business development and providing assistance to key clients who required my expertise.

CORPORATE WELLNESS PROGRAMMES

Couch to 5k with L&T Realty

Shrikant Joshi, CEO of L&T Realty, expressed a strong interest in our services and wanted to implement a corporate wellness programme for his employees. With the assistance of the Human Resources (HR) department, we launched the programme, 'Couch to 5k.' This initiative involved conducting fitness assessments and body composition analyses for all employees. We identified approximately 100 overweight employees with comorbidities to form a focus group that required special attention.

The 'Couch to 5k' programme spanned 45 days and encompassed nutrition, support and guidance. A nutritionist visited the employees every week to monitor their progress, while a trainer conducted 45-minute training sessions two to three times a week. To conclude the training, we organised a grand gala event. The day commenced at 6 a.m. with Zumba, warm-up exercises and a flag-off for a 5k run, which began and ended at L&T Realty's Powai office.

To ensure the safety and well-being of the participants, we had an ambulance, doctor, volunteers, guards and enthusiastic cheerleaders stationed along the route, providing water to the runners, many of whom were participating for the first time. After the programme, we awarded certificates to all participants and presented special trophies to the male and female winners.

The programme was an astounding success and left a lasting impression on the employees. The company witnessed a significant transformation in its workforce, with employees adopting healthier habits and prioritising their well-being.

Impressed by the programme's achievements, Mr Joshi announced a new challenge—a 10-kilometre run—and decided to extend the programme for an additional three months.

I had only 90 days to prepare him. So, he decided to hire a personal trainer from Virtus and consult with me for a nutrition plan. Nitin also started training his wife, Jyotsna, who was an athlete in school and college. It was wonderful to see the couple training together in the mornings and evenings, constantly pushing each other to improve.

Mr Joshi focused on developing endurance to run 10 kilometres without stopping. He worked out with Nitin in the mornings, gradually progressing from running 500 metres to completing the entire 10 kilometres without a break. Achieving this at the age of 65 filled him with pride.

He became leaner, with a lower body fat percentage and weight loss. Moreover, he gained flexibility and agility, allowing him to fit into his old clothes that didn't fit before. This experience reinforces my belief that obtaining an amazing body is merely a by-product of exercise and fitness.

As for Jyotsna Joshi, she followed a simple nutrition plan that seamlessly integrated into her lifestyle. The plan was designed so that they didn't have to prepare separate meals for each other or the rest of the family.

Nutrition plans should be easy to follow to ensure lifelong adherence. Even small modifications can have a significant impact when implemented correctly, as the journey towards health and fitness is a long-term process.

I am thrilled that they have embraced this philosophy and have been with us for five years.

NDTV-Nirmal Lifestyle Marks for Sports campaign

On 31 January 2010, we launched a personalised training programme for Dharmesh Jain and his family from the Nirmal Group. Within a year, they could observe the transformation in their weight levels and overall fitness. Their endurance and strength also increased, and the entire family gained knowledge about nutrition and healthy eating.

Dharmesh was so delighted with the results that he requested me to initiate a wellness programme for his employees, as he wanted fitness to be a top priority in his company. I began with nutrition consulting once a week and training his employees thrice a week, while Nitin would take care of the rest of the training.

Dharmesh then decided to take this a step further and wanted to organise a fitness movement to kindle fitness awareness among people, especially students. So, in 2013, partnering with NDTV, Nirmal Lifestyle launched the 'Fit India Movement', a first-of-its-kind long-term campaign to change the way India thinks about fitness and inspire us to become a healthier nation.

Mission 1 of the campaign was 'Marks for Sports', which aimed to develop fitter, more active and healthier lifestyles for the youth of today. The core belief of this campaign lay within the premise that if schools and, more importantly, different boards of education include Sports as a part of the main curriculum and allocate marks for it, then parents, as well as children, will devote more time to sports, setting them on the path of a lifetime of fitness. These marks will add to the student's overall percentage and performance in that academic year.

I liked the idea, and Dharmesh wanted me to be a part of the programme. We met up with school principals and launched the programme immediately. We organised fitness sessions for all age groups of kids and apprised them about healthy eating through interactive talk shows.

Dharmesh also launched the Marks for Sports Awards nights and roped in Ranbir Kapoor as the brand ambassador. A gala Awards night was held at ITC Maratha Sheraton in New Delhi—a night I will never forget for I could meet the legends of sports at that function like Sania Mirza, Milkha Singh and Mahesh Bhupathi. I was also surprised to receive the Lifetime Achievement Award in the 'Against the Odds' category.

I was extremely happy with this initiative, as it would lead to a generation of fit, healthy children who will take to sports because of their inclination and also for the marks allocated for it.

HIGH NET WORTH INDIVIDUALS (HNIS)

He grasped the nuance of nutrition

Rajkumar Hirani
Film director

Virtus's personal training business gained popularity through word-of-mouth publicity and referrals. One notable referral came from renowned film director **Rajkumar Hirani**, who was recommended to us by Dharmesh Jain.

I visited Mr Hirani at his home, and following our protocol, we began with a pathological test, fitness assessment and body composition analysis. We then introduced him to a comprehensive nutrition plan, followed by personal training sessions.

The training sessions commenced at 6.30 a.m. with one of my trainers, and within six months, Mr Hirani witnessed significant improvements in his endurance levels. Although his weight increased, his body fat percentage dropped. Moreover, his agility, strength and body mass all experienced noticeable enhancements. I provided him with weekly nutrition consultations for six months. We subsequently continued with a maintenance programme for an additional two years.

Mr Hirani grasped the importance of proper nutrition and has since maintained his health and fitness. Staying active is crucial, and individuals can choose any activity that brings them joy. Our greatest achievement lies in the fact that once the maintenance programme concludes, all our clients continue to lead a healthy lifestyle without deviation.

I consider myself truly fortunate to have crossed paths with such a humble individual. Mr Hirani even assisted me with this book by patiently listening to my story and referring me to a publisher. I am grateful to God for bringing such wonderful people into my life.

His best is yet to come

Vedaant Madhavan

International swimmer

With a lifelong interest in sports, I've always enjoyed training athletes. At Virtus, we've developed a comprehensive sports nutrition and training programme. This includes genetic testing, pathology tests to identify deficiencies in recovery factors like B12, Calcium and Vitamin D3, assessment of sports-specific fitness status, body composition analysis and a scientific post-training sports nutrition programme with a periodisation process.

Our clientele encompasses various age groups, but the notable one I'd like to mention is Vedaant Madhavan, the son of renowned actor R. Madhavan and his wife, Sarita. I've been guiding him in sports nutrition for several years now. In his case, we followed the entire process and protocol, starting from genetics to a Patola G Test, which helped us understand his fitness level, lifestyle, food choices, overall health and immunity. As an athlete striving to excel, he must remain injury-free and maintain optimal health.

Therefore, my role extended beyond managing his nutrition. I also ensured that he maintained a robust immune system, enabling him to give his best in competitions. Our association began in 2018, and within two years, he was ready to participate in national and international events. He broke numerous national records and has now qualified for the 2023 Commonwealth Games. While his achievements are impressive, I firmly believe that his best is yet to come.

In the realm of sports, many trainers tend to overload their athletes with unnecessary supplements, medications and even banned substances. I am aware of the detrimental effects of chemicals on our bodies. True performance can only be achieved when the body and mind are in good health, and harmful chemicals, whether in the form of supplements or drugs, are unnecessary.

Even after an athlete's prime, their health should not fail them, even if they are no longer actively involved in sports. Therefore, prioritising healthcare during the formative years is crucial. I feel a sense of responsibility in advising my clients on the right healthcare practices, knowing that once health is lost, its recovery is uncertain and time-consuming.

Age is merely a number

Jayesh Choksi

Founder, Choksi Vithaldas Rambhai

One of the 'youngest' clients I had the privilege to work with was Mr Jayesh Choksi, a renowned jeweller who embarked on his fitness journey at the age of 58. He was referred to Virtus to lead a healthy life and was willing to invest both time and money to regain his health.

From the outset, I made it clear that we do not endorse fad diets. I always advise my clients to commit to at least six months, as that's when the investment in our services, particularly in my role as a wellness coach, truly pays off. Mr Choksi chose this option, recognising the significant difference between hiring me as a dedicated guide and receiving personal training from one of our trainers.

After studying his eating habits and preferences, I devised a personalised nutrition plan for him, carefully considering the timing and portion sizes, and importantly, incorporating his favourite foods into the plan! Remarkably, within a month and a half, he shed five kilos and achieved a body fat percentage of three per cent.

With his nutrition on track, it was time to introduce him to our training programme. Initially, we went for short runs together, but it became evident that running wasn't his preferred activity. One day, we decided to run on a scenic track within the beautiful Sanjay Gandhi National Park in Borivali, and he discovered genuine enjoyment in that experience. It was a turning point for us both, as I knew that if he found pleasure in an activity, he would be motivated to continue it for life.

This embodies our philosophy—whether it's nutrition, physical activity, or training programmes, we strive for our clients to find joy in them, transforming these practices into sustainable lifestyles that extend beyond a few months.

From that point onward, there was no looking back for Jayesh Choksi. With the guidance of one of Virtus's trainers, Roshan Ghanekar, he underwent mountaineering training and accomplished successful ascents of Mount Kilimanjaro and Mount Elbrus within two years. Currently, at the age of 61, he is relentlessly training to conquer Mount Everest. He is a shining example, proving that age is merely a number.

CONCLUSION

In the tapestry of life, the laughter we enjoy and the tears we shed hold a significance beyond what meets the eye. They are not random occurrences, but rather intricately woven threads that connect us to our mortality. It is a realisation that has been etched into the core of my being through the trials and tribulations of my journey. Our breath, our very existence, is a delicate calculation that often goes unnoticed. Yet, in the ebb and flow of life, it is vital to remain cognizant of this truth.

When happiness graces our lives and when smiles illuminate our faces, it becomes our duty to approach these moments with humility and kindness. During such times, we possess the power to become conduits of compassion, spreading warmth through kind words, thoughtful actions, or even the simplest of deeds. This responsibility weighs heavy upon us, for we know not when life's tides may turn, plunging us into the depths of darkness.

It is in those moments of despair that our acts of kindness shine the brightest. Those whose lives we have touched, who have witnessed the tenderness of our souls, step forward as guardian angels. They become the pillars of strength, enveloping us in their protective embrace. Their unwavering support and unwarranted benevolence become our sanctuary, a light that guides us through the abyss. We learn that the bonds we forge through selflessness are the ones that sustain us in our darkest hours.

For me, the battle against cancer has become the ultimate human race. It is a marathon that tests not only the limits of our physical endurance but also the depths of our spirit. It is a race that unites individuals from all walks of life, their hearts beating in unison, fuelled by hope and resilience. In this race, we find ourselves pushing beyond our perceived boundaries, running with unwavering determination towards an intangible finish line.

Through the trials and tribulations of this fight, I have come to understand the true meaning of comradeship. It transcends the mere camaraderie found in athletic pursuits; it embodies the essence of what it means to be human. It is a bond forged through shared struggles, a support system that knows no bounds. In the face of adversity, we discover the profound strength that lies within the collective.

This battle against cancer, this ultimate human race, is not one that can be fought in isolation. It requires the unwavering support of those around us—friends, family, and even strangers who have been touched by our story. Together, we form an indomitable force, ready to tackle the challenges that lie ahead. It is through this unity that we find solace and inspiration, propelling us forward even when the odds seem insurmountable.

As I reflect upon my journey, I am filled with gratitude for the lessons learned and the connections made, and filled with a renewed sense of purpose. Comrades, the ultimate humane race, has taught me that our journey is not defined by the battles we face, but rather by the love and compassion we extend along the way. It is in the smallest gestures, the gentlest words, that we leave an indelible mark on the world.

May we all strive to run this race with open hearts, knowing that our actions ripple through the lives of others. Together, let us paint a tapestry of kindness, love, and unwavering support, for it is in these threads that we find our strength, our humanity, and our ultimate triumph.

–Shiraz Siddiqui

ACKNOWLEDGEMENTS

This book is dedicated to my parents, who have shown unwavering love and belief in me. They will forever hold a special place in my heart.

It has been a challenging nineteen-year-old battle with cancer, during which time, my friends, family and clients continuously urged me to chronicle my life story. When I reflect on my childhood as a youngster who used to evade studies, the idea of writing a book seemed unimaginable. However, once I decided to do it, the process of sharing my life journey unravelled automatically and proved to be an incredibly unique experience.

As a professional nutritionist and wellness coach, I have always aspired to assist newly diagnosed cancer patients, helping them understand the significance of nutrition, staying active and maintaining a positive mindset. Recognising the difficulties in reaching a wider audience, I decided to share my life's struggles through this book.

It is my earnest endeavour to inspire and motivate not only cancer patients but also anyone who refuses to relinquish hope in the face of adversity. Cancer, in my perspective, is simply a word that I transform into 'CAN, SIR.'

A battle cannot be fought alone; hence, I am immensely grateful to the numerous individuals who have aided me in every aspect of my life. At the outset, I extend my heartfelt appreciation to Dr Abhay Bhave, who has been my guiding light, confidante and dear friend since my diagnosis in 2004. His unwavering dedication, discipline and positive outlook are truly remarkable. Dr Bhave is akin to family, and I am overjoyed that I was able to inspire him to embrace nutrition and fitness training, not only for himself but also for his loved ones.

I am grateful to Dr Shashikant Apte, Dr Aditi and the entire haematology team at Sahyadri Hospital in Pune, where I underwent my bone marrow transplant. Dr Apte's exceptional expertise in this field has been invaluable.

Coming from a lower middle-class family background, financing the exorbitant costs of cancer treatment presented a significant challenge. However, with the grace of the Almighty, I was blessed to have in my life many people who came to my aid during life's most arduous phase. This book would be incomplete without acknowledging each one of them. I extend my sincere thanks to Sadanand Shetty, Gautam Jasra, Pankaj Rajdhan, Shamsu Lalani, Ankit Agarwal, Mahrukh Khan, Sanjeev Mansotra, Dharmesh Jain, Rajiv Jain, Nainesh and Jesal Shah, Dhananjay and Poonam Sandhu, Subodh Menon, Shrikant Joshi, Praful Mungi, Sagar Rajukumar Desai, Rashmin Rughani, Ajay Ashar, Niraj and Alpa Shah, Farah Khan, Dipesh Gindra, Nitij Arenja, Kausar Ladha, Manju and Nazia.

I am immensely grateful to Ajay Arora and his family, who not only provided me with financial and emotional support but also embraced me as a member of their own family. I consider myself truly blessed to have such an individual in my life.

During my initial cancer diagnosis, I was fortunate to have empathetic colleagues at work who were aware of the post-treatment complications I faced and allowed me to work reduced hours. I extend my gratitude to Dr Kalpana, who has been with me from the time of diagnosis until now, and to everyone at JW Marriott Hotel, Juhu. This is the place where I found friends who have become like family and who continue to stay in touch.

I extend a special thanks to Rajkumar Hirani and Manjeet, who assisted me in finding the right publisher and inspired me to write this book. I would also like to mention Ashishwang Godha, who provided invaluable support in the writing process, and R. Sridhar, who edited the book.

I express my heartfelt appreciation to the entire team at Virtus, which has been my pillar of strength. My teammates have supported me throughout my journey, from the inception of Virtus to battling cancer, believing in me, and standing by my side when I needed them the most. I am incredibly grateful to have such an amazing team.

My gratitude extends eternally to my incredible wife, Nida, who entered my life like a guardian angel during my weakest moments. Without her unwavering support, I would not have been able to complete this book. She is not just my wife but also my best friend, the person I always yearned for, and I will forever be grateful to God for bringing her into my life.

Last, but not the least, I would like to extend my thanks to Vikas Rakheja, Rashmi Menon, Bidisha Srivastava and Sanika Shendye Kher from Manjul Publishing House.

ABOUT THE AUTHOR

Mumbai-born **Shiraz Siddiqui** (1976–2023) was a fitness instructor and marathon runner. His passion to see every person, young and old, fit and healthy in life, is what drove him to start his own fitness consultancy company Virtus Wellness Pvt. Ltd. in April 2010. At Virtus, he guided his clients towards healthier lives. Shiraz fought cancer four times and was one of the rare people who dealt with two types of cancer in his lifetime. He passed away in 2023.

Although he is not with us today, his legacy lives on in the hearts and minds of all who were associated with him.